*Pocket Guide
to Herbal
Remedies*

Pocket Guide to Herbal Remedies

Lane P. Johnson, MD, MPH

Associate Professor, Clinical Family and Community Medicine

University of Arizona College of Medicine

Tucson, Arizona

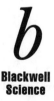

**Blackwell
Science**

Blackwell Science, Inc.
© 2002 by Lane Johnson

Editorial Offices:
Commerce Place, 350 Main Street, Malden, Massachusetts 02148, USA
Osney Mead, Oxford OX2 0EL, England
25 John Street, London WC1N 2BS, England
23 Ainslie Place, Edinburgh EH3 6AJ, Scotland
54 University Street, Carlton, Victoria 3053, Australia

Other Editorial Offices:
Blackwell Wissenschafts-Verlag GmbH, Kurfürstendamm 57,
    10707 Berlin, Germany
Blackwell Science KK, MG Kodenmacho Building, 7-10 Kodenmacho
    Nihombashi, Chuo-ku, Tokyo 104, Japan
Iowa State University Press, A Blackwell Science Company,
    2121 S. State Avenue, Ames, Iowa 50014-8300, USA

Distributors:
The Americas
    Blackwell Publishing   telephone orders:
    c/o AIDC   800–216–252
    P.O. Box 20   fax orders:
    50 Winter Sport Lane   802–864–7626
    Williston, VT 05495-0020

Australia   telephone orders:
    Blackwell Science Pty, Ltd.   03–9347–0300
    54 University Street   fax orders:
    Carlton, Victoria 3053   03–9349–3016

Outside The Americas and Australia
    Blackwell Science, Ltd.   telephone orders:
    c/o Marston Book Services, Ltd.   44–01235–465500
    P.O. Box 269   fax orders:
    Abingdon   44–01235–465555
    Oxon OX14 4YN England

Acquisitions: Beverly Copland
Development: Amy Nuttbrock
Production: Irene Herlihy
Manufacturing: Lisa Flanagan
Marketing Manager: Toni Fournier
Design and typesetting: Boynton Hue Studio

Printed and bound by Sheridan Books

Printed in the United States of America

02 03 04 05 5 4 3 2

The Blackwell Science logo is a trade mark of Blackwell Science Ltd.,
registered at the United Kingdom Trade Marks Registry

To my grandmother Mona Warfield,
who, at 100 years of age, continues to be
a shining beacon of unconditional love

*C*ontents

Preface

This book is designed as a quick reference for primary care clinicians, physicians, nurse practitioners, physician assistants, residents and medical students, nurses, and the general public.

It is intended to be a pocket reference to review indications, dosages, contraindications, and interactions of commonly used herbal remedies that patients may be taking. Its secondary purpose is as a convenient consumer guide for most of the herbal remedies that one's friends and family might be taking, not knowing if there could be a drug interaction or adverse effect.

This pocket guide covers most of the herbal remedies and clinical issues that primary care clinicians will commonly encounter in their practices. It is hoped that by having an easily accessible source of medically sound information about herbs, clinicians will be more willing and able to engage in a conversation with their patients about these products.

Recent studies suggest that in the United States, over 15 million adults utilize herbal remedies during a given year. A majority of these patients also utilize standard medical care for the same problem; over 30% do not disclose the use of alternative therapies to their physicians.

Being familiar with the over 4000 drugs listed in the Physicians Desk Reference is daunting enough to clinical practitioners, but having to consider another 700+ herbal products is even more overwhelming. Given standard medicine's skepticism of alternative therapies, it is not surprising that patients and their clinicians have engaged in a medical version of "don't ask, don't tell."

Herbal products are often advertised as natural and safe. While severe reactions to herbal remedies are rare, the increased use of herbs has resulted in an increased number of significant reactions and interactions with other substances. The rapidly growing number of journal articles and textbooks on this topic attest to the need for clinicians to pay more attention to the issues of herbal treatment.

In my own practice, I make a point of asking patients which herbs and supplements they take. As they list each one, I question why they are taking it. Frequently, they are not sure. It may have been recommended by an acquaintance, or more often, a clerk at the health food store. I then ask the patient if the product is helping. Again, patients are often not sure. In those instances, I recommend they discontinue the product, suggesting they can restart the product if they feel worse. Patients are usually happy to stop.

What most patients really want from their clinicians is an honest dialog about their therapeutic options. In some cases, herbal therapies are as efficacious as the standard treatments we might normally offer. Many times they are not. In general, I find most patients when given the options make good choices. Having readily available information regarding herbal remedies enhances our ability to offer appropriate choices to our patients.

*A*cknowledgments

Many thanks to my family, Susan, Danny, and Cassidy, who will be glad to get the dining room table, and my evenings, back. I bow to my medical mentors Larry Moher and Doug Lindsey, who taught me to keep it simple. A nod to Andy Weil and Michael Moore, for feeding my herbal appetite. Thanks to Liz, Carol, Irma, and Stephanie, the CUP house Crewe, for their ongoing encouragement, and to Susan, Ron, and Tracy from the International Health Class for pulling me (oh-so reluctantly) back on stage each year. A hearty pat on the back to Rich Rivera, my research assistant, and Catharine "Kiki" Riley, my editorial assistant. A tot o' grog to Bev and Amy at Blackwell Science, who found my ship, hunted me down, made me draw the map, and then take them to dig up the treasure. I owe lunch to my friends and colleagues Jim Kerwin, Mark Bessette, Molly Roberts, Steve Menhennett, Ed Schwager, Ramesh Karra, Mark Rogers, Steve Galper, and Richard "Buck" Hendrix, for taking the manuscript for a test drive. Give the glory to them and the blame to me. I have been honored by, and am grateful to, the patients and students who have walked the path with me. The plant world, and my little spot in the Sonoran Desert, continue to entrance and enrich me. Happy trails to all.

LPJ
Tucson
April 2001

*A*bout the Author

Lane P. Johnson, MD, MPH is an Associate Professor of Clinical Family and Community Medicine at the University of Arizona College of Medicine. He has over 15 years of clinical experience in both rural and urban settings. His practice has included consultation in alternative therapies and acupuncture. He has lectured widely on these subjects to a variety of professional and consumer audiences.

*A*bout this Book

Why herbal remedies? Herbs are rarely prescribed by clinicians; more often, herbs are self-prescribed by patients, or recommended by friends, acquaintances, or health food store clerks. This is similar to the use of over-the-counter remedies, which are also generally self-prescribed. The term *remedy* suggests greater involvement on the part of the patient in the utilization of the product; in most cases, the clinician may be more advisor than prescriber. Like over-the-counter remedies, herbal products are subject to advertising claims of efficacy and safety, and there is potential for abuse without objective medical counsel.

Research into herbal products is progressing so rapidly that any book is a snapshot of what is known at that point in time. Most herbs, sadly, remain poorly studied, if at all. Those studies that do exist are often of poor quality, and results not necessarily applicable to large populations. Contraindications to herbal therapies and interaction with medicines are just beginning to be recognized and written about in medical literature.

The situation is further complicated by the classification of herbal products as food supplements rather than medication. Vague claims can be made for therapeutic efficacy and safety without substantiation. Moreover, labeling of herbal products can also be misleading. Unlike medications, there is no guarantee that what is listed on the bottle is what is in the bottle, or is at a dosage that is even remotely therapeutic. It is not known if the herb sat in the field, the storehouse, the manufacturer's shelves, the delivery truck, or the store shelf for so long as to be rendered useless. The best one can do is to recommend national brands with expiration dates and labels that certify a specific dosage of the active ingredient. Several drug companies have been toying with pharmaceutical grade herbal products, but they are generally too expensive for most people.

What we have attempted to accomplish with this book is a review of the best books and articles synthesized into a clinically useful format. The resources consulted are listed in the References section.

Disclaimer

Every effort has been made to provide a clinical pocket guide to herbal remedies that is as accurate, complete, and concise as possible. The field of herbal remedies is rapidly changing. Any effort is a snapshot in time, and is out of date as soon as the writing is done. At this time, there is more unknown about herbal remedies than is known. Differences within and among plant species, manufacturers, distributors, clinicians, and patients make it impossible to predict a specific reaction to a specific remedy at a specific dosage in a specific patient at a specific time. The Author and the Publisher make no claims for the efficacy or safety of any information published in this guide. The risk lies entirely with the reader, dispenser, and consumer of herbal remedies.

Template

The following template is used to describe each herb.
An explanation follows the example:

Ginkgo biloba
Ginkgo, kew tree, maidenhair tree

Principal reported indication(s):
Dementia *** +/−
Intermittent claudication ** +/−
Memory loss *
Raynaud's disease
Tinnitis *
Vertigo **

Probable effective dosage:
120–240 mg 2–3 times daily

Contraindications:
Anti-thrombotic agents

Potential adverse reactions:
Allergic reaction
Bleeding
Dyspepsia/nausea

Potential medication interactions:
Antithrombotic agents

Comments:
None

Explanation of Template

Scientific Name
Genus (capitalized) and species (not capitalized) are
listed in italics. If more than two species have similar
effects, the scientific name is listed as *Genus spp.*

Common Name(s)
The most frequently used common name is listed first. Other common names are listed in alphabetical order. Common names are indexed in the back of the book.

Other names
Synonymous scientific names are printed in italics and listed in alphabetical order. They are indexed in the back of the book.

Principal reported indication(s)
Principal reported indications are listed in alphabetical order and by efficacy. The number of stars gives a rating system of human trials:

No stars	Unproven, historical use, or indication without support.
*	Anecdotal support, or a few human case studies.
**	One or more human studies that demonstrate some efficacy for the indication. Trials may not have been randomized, may not have control groups, or may not have large numbers of subjects.
***	At least one large randomized controlled human study of demonstrated efficacy.
+/–	Indicates inconsistent results of efficacy in clinical trials

Principal reported indications are indexed in the back of the book.

Probable effective dosage
Effective dosage, if known. Many herbal preparations may not have effective amounts of an herb for a variety of reasons discussed in the introduction.

Contraindications

Conditions or situations in which the herbal remedy should not be used. Listed in alphabetical order and indexed in the back of the book. Avoidance of use of herbal remedies in children, during lactation, or pregnancy is listed when that specific contraindication is substantiated in reference texts. Use of herbal remedies in any of these situations must be carefully weighed against the risk.

Potential adverse reactions

Listed in alphabetical order.

Potential medication interactions:

Medication interactions are listed as noted in references. They are listed in alphabetical order and indexed in the back of the book. Theoretical interactions have not been included, although several reference texts include them.

Comments:

As appropriate.

Most Effective Remedies

A pharmacology colleague once reported that most physicians use a total of 30 herbs about 95% of the time. The most effective herbal remedies (based on human studies) are listed below with their indications.

Aesculus hippocastanum
    Chronic venous insufficiency ***

Allium sativum
    Hyperlipidemia *** +/–

Arctostaphylos spp.
    Urinary tract infection **

Borago officinalis
    Rheumatic disorders **

Capsicum spp.
    Herpes zoster (shingles) ** (topical)

Cassia spp.
    Constipation ***

Centella asiatica
    Chronic venous insufficiency **
    Hypertension **

Cetraria islandica
    Bronchitis **
    Laryngitis **

Cimicifuga racemosa
    Climacteric symptoms ***

Commiphora mukul
    Hypercholesterolemia **

Crataegus monogyra
    Congestive heart failure ***

Cucurbita pepo
  Benign prostatic hypertrophy ** +/−

Curcuma longa
  Dyspepsia **

Cynaria scolymus
  Dyspepsia **

Echinacea spp.
  Immune stimulation **

Ginkgo biloba
  Dementia *** +/−

Glycine spp. *
  Hypercholesterolemia ***

Glycyrrhiza glabra
  Peptic ulcer **

Humulus lupulus
  Insomnia**

Hypericum perforatum
  Depression *** +/−

Linum usitatissimum
  Hypercholesterolemia **

Melaleuca alternifolia
  Tinia pedis **

Mentha piperita
  Dyspepsia **
  Intestinal spasm **
  Irritable bowel syndrome **

Oenothera spp.
  Premenstrual syndrome ***
  Rheumatic disorders **

Pausinystalia yohimbe
  Erectile dysfunction **

Panax ginseng
   Stress tonic **

Piper methysticum
   Anxiety **

Plantago spp.
   Constipation **
   Hypercholesterolemia **
   Irritable bowel syndrome **

Pygeum africanum
   Benign prostatic hypertrophy ***

Salvia officinalis
   Hyperhydrosis **

Serenoa repens
   Benign prostatic hypertrophy ***

Tanacetum parthenium
   Migraine prophylaxis ***

Trifolium pratense
   Benign prostatic hypertrophy **

Trigonella foenum-graecum
   Hypercholesterolemia ***

Urtica spp.
   Benign prostatic hypertrophy **

Vaccinium macrocarpon
   Urinary tract infection prevention **

Valerian spp.
   Insomnia **

Vitis vinifera
   Chronic venous insufficiency **

Zingiber officinale
   Nausea ** +/−
   Motion sickness **

*A*chillea millefolium

Yarrow, milfoil, nosebleed plant, plumajillo, wound wort

Principal reported indication(s):
Dyspepsia/nausea
Fever
Hypertension
Irritable bowel syndrome
Menorrhagia
Wound healing

Probable effective dosage:
2–4 grams as tea 3 times daily
5 mL tincture 3 times daily

Contraindications:
Allergy to plants of the Compositae family
Pregnancy

Potential adverse reactions:
Allergic reaction
Photosensitivity

Potential medication interactions:
No significant medication interactions have been noted

Comments:
None

Actaea spp.

White cohosh, baneberry, bugbane, herb
Christopher, toad root

Principal reported indication(s):
Amenorrhea
Emetic
Constipation

Probable effective dosage:
No dosage noted

Contraindications:
Gastritis
Gastric or duodenal ulcer
Inflammatory bowel disease
Lactation
Pregnancy

Potential adverse reactions:
Bloody diarrhea
Dyspepsia/nausea
Headache
Dermatitis/blistering (topical)
Palpitations

Potential medication interactions:
No significant medication interactions noted

Comments:
▶ *Actaea* has significant potential toxicity and should
not be used internally.

*A*esculus hippocastanum

Horse chestnut, buckeye, chestnut, common horse chestnut, Spanish chestnut

Principal reported indication(s):
Chronic venous insufficiency ***
Inflammation
Varicosities (topical)

Probable effective dosage:
250 mg standardized extract 1–3 times daily
1–4 mL tincture 3 times daily
1–2% gel applied topically several times daily

Contraindications:
Antithrombotic agents
Hepatic disorders
Lactation
Pregnancy
Renal disorders

Potential adverse reactions:
Allergic reaction
Dyspepsia/nausea/vomiting
Hepatotoxicity
Nephrotoxicity
Urticaria

Potential medication interactions:
Antithrombotic agents

Comments:
◗ The flower has significant potential toxicity and should not be used. Standardized extracts are made from seeds.

Agrimonia eupatoria

Agrimony, cockleburr, church steeples, common agrimony, sticklewort, stickwort

Principal reported indication(s):
Dermatitis (topical)
Diarrhea
Stomatitis/pharyngitis

Probable effective dosage:
3–6 grams herb as tea daily in divided doses
Poultice topically 2–3 times daily

Contraindications:
Cardiac disorders

Potential adverse reactions:
Hypotension (large doses)
Photodermatitis

Potential medication interactions:
Hypertensive drugs—may have increased effects.

Comments:
None

Allium cepa

Onion, green onion

Principal reported indication(s):
Anorexia
Arteriosclerosis
Bronchitis/cough
Dyspepsia
Hypercoagulability
Hyperlipidemia *
Hypertension
Upper respiratory infection

Probable effective dosage:
50 grams of fresh onion or 20 grams of dried onion daily

Contraindications:
No significant contraindications noted

Potential adverse reactions:
Allergic reaction
Dyspepsia
Dermatitis

Potential medication interactions:
Aspirin—may increase risk of allergic reaction.

Comments:
◗ Cooking may destroy therapeutic effect.

*A*llium sativum

Garlic, ajo, poor man's treacle, stinking rose

Principal reported indication(s):
Arteriosclerosis *
Bacterial infection
Hyperlipidemia *** +/−
Hypertension +/−
Viral infection

Probable effective dosage:
1 clove or ~1000 mg a day in 2 or 3 doses

Contraindications:
Antithrombotic drugs
Lactation

Potential adverse reactions:
Dyspepsia/nausea
Bleeding
Burns

Potential medication interactions:
Antithrombotic drugs—may increase effects.

Comments:
◗ Cooking may destroy therapeutic effect.
◗ Dried garlic capsules are likely as effective.

A *loe spp.*

Aloe, Barbados aloe, cape aloe

Principal reported indication(s):
Burns (topical)
Constipation
Dermatitis (topical)
Wound healing (topical)

Probable effective dosage:
Gel applied topically 4–5 times daily
50–200 mg caps daily (internally)

Contraindications:
Allergic reaction to plants of Lilliaceae family
Bowel obstruction (internal)
Lactation (internal)
Pregnancy (internal)
Intestinal disorders (internal)

Potential adverse reactions:
Allergic reaction
Intestinal obstruction (internal)
Electrolyte or mineral depletion (internal)

Potential medication interactions:
No significant medication interactions noted

Comments:
▶ Internal use is not recommended.
▶ Internal use may cause urine to turn red.

*A*lthea officinalis

Marshmallow, mortification root, sweetweed

Principal reported indication(s):
Bronchitis/cough
Irritable bowel syndrome
Nausea/vomiting
Pharyngitis
Wound healing

Probable effective dosage:
5–6 grams as tea daily in divided doses

Contraindications:
No significant contraindications noted

Potential adverse reactions:
No significant adverse reactions noted

Potential medication interactions:
Oral drugs—may delay absorption of other drugs.

Comments:
None

*A*maranthus spp.

Amaranth, lady bleeding, love-lies-bleeding, pigweed, pilewort, prince's feather, red cockscomb, velvet flower

Principal reported indication(s):
Diarrhea
Gastric ulcers
Stomatitis/pharyngitis

Probable effective dosage:
1 tsp in one cup of cold water 1–2 times daily
1 tsp tincture 1–2 times daily

Contraindications:
No significant contraindications noted

Potential adverse reactions:
No significant adverse effects noted

Potential medication interactions:
No significant medication interactions noted

Comments:
None

Ananas comosus

Pineapple, bromilian, pineapple enzyme

Principal reported indication(s):
Cancer adjuvant
Dysmenorrhea
Inflammation
Wound healing

Probable effective dosage:
80–500 mg of bromilian extract 2–3 times daily

Contraindications:
Allergic reaction
Antithrombotic drugs

Potential adverse reactions:
Allergic reaction
Dyspepsia/nausea

Potential medication interactions:
Antithrombotic drugs—may increase effects.
Tetracycline—levels may be increased.

Comments:
None

*A**nethum graveolens*

Dill, American dill, dill weed, dilly, European dill

Principal reported indication(s):
Dyspepsia
Flatulence
Galactagogue
Intestinal spasm
Insomnia

Probable effective dosage:
3 grams of seeds daily
1–3 grams herb as tea 3 times daily
0.1–0.3 grams essential oil daily in divided doses

Contraindications:
No significant contraindications noted

Potential adverse reactions:
Allergic reaction
Dermatitis

Potential medication interactions:
No significant medication interactions noted

Comments:
None

*A*ngelica archangelica

Angelica, European angelica, garden angelica, wild angelica, *Archangelica officinalis*

Principal reported indication(s):
Anorexia
Flatulence
Intestinal spasm

Probable effective dosage:
1–2 grams herb as tea 2–3 times daily

Contraindications:
Antithrombotic drugs

Potential adverse reactions:
Photosensitivity

Potential medication interactions:
Photosensitizing drugs—may increase effects.
Antithrombotic drugs—may increase effects.

Comments:
None

*A*ngelica sinensis
Dong quai, Chinese angelica

Principal reported indication(s):
Climacteric symptoms
Premenstrual syndrome
Dysmenorrhea

Probable effective dosage:
1–2 grams as tea or capsules 3 times daily

Contraindications:
Antithrombotic therapy
Lactation
Pregnancy

Potential adverse reactions:
Photosensitization

Potential medication interactions:
Antithrombotic agents—may increase effects.

Comments:
None

A*nthemis nobilis*

Chamomile, common chamomile, English chamomile, ground apple, Roman chamomile, *Chamaemelum nobile*

Principal reported indication(s):
Anxiety
Dyspepsia/nausea
Insomnia
Irritable bowel disease
Dysmenorrhea

Probable effective dosage:
1–3 grams as tea several times daily

Contraindications:
Allergy to plants of the Compositae family
Pregnancy

Potential adverse reactions:
Allergic reaction

Potential medication interactions:
No significant medical interactions noted

Comments:
None

*A*rctium lappa

Burdock, bardana, beggar's buttons, cockle buttons, clotbur, edible burdock, great burdock, great burr, hardock, lappa, love leaves, personata, phlanthropium, thorny burr

Principal reported indication(s):
Dyspepsia/nausea
Eczema
Edema
Fever
Urticaria (topical)

Probable effective dosage:
2 grams root as tea 3–4 times daily
Essential oil topically several times daily

Contraindications:
Pregnancy

Potential adverse reactions:
Dermatitis (topical)

Potential medication interactions:
No significant medication interactions noted

Comments:
▶ Some commercial preparations have been contaminated with atropine.

Arctostaphylos spp.

Urva ursi, bear berry, bear grape, hog berry, kinikinik, madrone, manzanilla, manzanita

Principal reported indication(s):
Edema
Urinary tract inflammation (antiseptic) **

Probable effective dosage:
3–4 grams as tea up to 4 times daily

Contraindications:
Children < 12 years
Lactation
Pregnancy
Renal disorders

Potential adverse reactions:
Dyspepsia/nausea
Toxic reactions have occurred in very large doses,
   including nausea, vomiting, collapse and death.
Urine may turn green.

Potential medication interactions:
Drugs that cause acidic urine will decrease effectiveness
   of herb.

Comments:
None

*A*rmoracia rusticana

Horseradish, pepperrot, *Cochlearia armoracia*

Principal reported indication(s):
Edema
Rheumatic disorders (topical)
Upper respiratory infection
Urinary tract infection

Probable effective dosage:
2–4 grams fresh root before meals

Contraindications:
Children < 4 years
Renal disorder
Stomach or duodenal ulcers

Potential adverse reactions:
Allergic reaction
Diarrhea (in large doses)
Mucus membrane irritation
Vomiting (in large doses)

Potential medication interactions:
Anticholinergic drugs—may reduce effects.
Cholinergic drugs—may increase effects.

Comments:
❱ Should only be used in quantities used in flavoring.

Arnica montana

Arnica, leopard's bane, mountain daisy,
mountain snuff, mountain tobacco,
sneezewort, wolf's bane

Principal reported indication(s):
Acne/boils (topical)
Sprains/strains/bruising (topical)

Probable effective dosage:
20–25% ointment or tincture topically twice a day.
   Should not be used internally.

Contraindications:
Allergy to herb
Children < 12 years
Internal use
Open wounds

Potential adverse reactions:
Allergic reaction
Dermatitis
Dyspepsia, nausea, vomiting (internal use)
Hepatotoxicity (internal use)

Potential medication interactions:
No significant medication interactions noted

Comments:
▶ Should not be taken internally.

Artemisia spp.

Wormwood, absinth, common wormwood, mugwort, green ginger, Chinese wormwood, sweet wormwood, sweet Annie

Principal reported indication(s):
Anorexia
Anxiety
Biliary disorders
Dyspepsia
Hepatic disorder
Insomnia
Wound healing (topical)

Probable effective dosage:
2–3 grams herb as tea 2–3 times daily

Contraindications:
Pregnancy

Potential adverse reactions:
Allergic reaction
CNS depression
Cramps
Dizziness
Hallucinations
Headache
Vomiting
Toxic reactions have occurred, especially with tincture of *Artemisia absinthium,* an alcoholic beverage.

Potential medication interactions:
Seizure drugs—may decrease effects.

Comments:
◗ *Artemisia* has significant potential toxicity and is not recommended.

Asclepias spp.

Milkweed, blood flower, butterfly milkweed, Canada root, flux root, orange milkweed, pleurisy root, swallowwort, swamp milkweed, tuber root, white root, wind root

Principal reported indication(s):
Asthma
Bronchitis/cough
Fever
Intestinal spasm

Probable effective dosage:
No dosage noted

Contraindications:
Cardiac disorders
Lactation
Pregnancy

Potential adverse reactions:
Cardiotoxicity (high doses)
Dermatitis
Vomiting (high doses)

Potential medication interactions:
Cardiac glycoside drugs—may increase effects.

Comments:
▶ Use of *Asclepias* is not recommended.

Astragalus spp.

Milk vetch, Bei Qi, Huang-qi, membranous milk vetch, Mongolian milk vetch, tragacanth

Principal reported indication(s):
Fatigue
Immune stimulant *
Influenza
Ischemic heart failure *
Leukopenia *
Upper respiratory infections
Weakness

Probable effective dosage:
2–6 grams root daily
Two 250 mg capsules 3 times daily

Contraindications:
Antithrombotic drugs
Autoimmune disorders
Immunosuppressive drugs
Organ transplant recipients

Potential adverse reactions:
Immunosuppression (high doses)
Neurologic dysfunction due to selenium content

Potential medication interactions:
Antithrombotic drugs—may increase effects.
Immunosuppressive drugs—may increase or decrease
    effects.

Comments:
None

Avena sativa

Oats, haver, havercorn, haws, oat beard, oatmeal

Principal reported indication(s):
Dermatitis
Diabetes *
Eczema (topical)
Gout
Hyperlipidemia * +/−
Seborrhea
Warts

Probable effective dosage:
50–100 grams daily for cholesterol
1 cup as mash 1–2 times daily

Contraindications:
Celiac disease
Bowel obstruction

Potential adverse reactions:
Bloating/flatulence
Dermatitis

Potential medication interactions:
No significant medication interactions noted

Comments:
▶ Recent studies have demonstrated *Avena* is not effective in reducing the risk of colon cancer.

*B*arosma spp.

Buchu, diosma, honey, buchu, mountain buchu, round buchu, short buchu, short-leaved buchu

Principal reported indication(s):
Bladder inflammation
Edema
Urinary disinfectant
Urinary tract infection

Probable effective dosage:
1–2 grams daily

Contraindications:
Hepatic disorders
Pregnancy
Renal disorders

Potential adverse reactions:
Dyspepsia/nausea (essential oil)
Hepatic toxicity (essential oil)
Local irritation (essential oil)

Potential medication interactions:
No significant medication interactions noted

Comments:
▶ Toxicity has occurred with essential oil; use of the essential oil is not recommended.

*B*erberis spp.

Barberry, berberry, European barberry, jaundice berry, mountain grape, Oregon grape root, pepperidge bush, sow berry, sour spine, trailing mahonia, wood sour, *Mahonia spp.*

Principal reported indication(s):
Anorexia
Bronchitis/cough
Constipation
Diarrhea +/−
Dyspepsia
Intestinal spasm
Psoriasis * +/− (topical)

Probable effective dosage:
2 grams as tea daily
20–40 drops tincture daily

Contraindications:
Pregnancy
Renal disorders

Potential adverse reactions:
Allergic reaction
CNS disturbances (large doses)
Dermatitis (topical)
Diarrhea (large doses)
Renal irritation (large doses)
Vomiting (large doses)

Potential medication interactions:
No significant medication interactions noted

Comments:
▶ Toxic reactions have occurred from Berberine, a con-
stituent extracted from *Berberis spp.*
▶ *Berberis* is used as a substitute for *Hydrastis canadensis,* which is rapidly disappearing in the wild.

Bidens spp.

Burr marigold, water agrimony

Principal reported indication(s):
Alopecia
Colitis
Edema
Fever
Gout
Inflammation

Probable effective dosage:
No dosage noted

Contraindications:
No significant contraindications noted

Potential adverse reactions:
No adverse reactions noted

Potential medication interactions:
No medication interactions noted

Comments:
None

B*orago officinalis*

Borage, bee bread, borage seed oil, common borage, common bugloss, ox's tongue, starflower

Principal reported indication(s):
Bronchitis/cough
Depression
Galactagogue
Rheumatic disorders **
Upper respiratory infection

Probable effective dosage:
1.1–1.4 grams of borage seed oil daily

Contraindications:
Hepatic disorders
Phenothiazine drugs

Potential adverse reactions:
Constipation
Hepatotoxicity
Toxic reaction (large doses)

Potential medication interactions:
Phenothiazine drugs—increased seizure risk.

Comments:
▶ Arthritis treatment was by use of gamma-linolenic acid (GLA) derived from borage seed oil.

Calendula officinalis

Marigold, garden marigold, gold bloom, holly gold, Mary bud, pot marigold, poet's marigold

Principal reported indication(s):
Acne (topical)
Burns (topical)
Dermatitis (topical)
Eczema (topical)
Fungal infection (topical)
Gastric ulcers
Psoriasis
Skin ulcers (topical)
Stomatitis/pharyngitis (topical)
Wound healing

Probable effective dosage:
1 gram whole flower daily
5–10 mL tincture daily
Ointment or tincture topically several times a day

Contraindications:
Allergic reaction (rare)
Pregnancy (internally)

Potential adverse reactions:
Allergic reaction

Potential medication interactions:
No significant medication interactions noted

Comments:
None

Camellia sinensis

Green tea, chai, Chinese tea, matsu sha

Principal reported indication(s):
Cancer prevention * (large doses)
Dental caries *
Depression
Fatigue
Hypercholesterolemia (large doses) * +/−

Probable effective dosage:
2 grams herb as tea 4 or more times daily

Contraindications:
Children
Gastritis
Lactation
Pregnancy (over 5 cups daily)

Potential adverse reactions:
Allergic reaction
Anxiety
Gastritis
Hepatotoxicity (in chronic large doses)
Decreased iron metabolism (in children)
Insomnia
Tachycardia

Potential medication interactions:
Alkaline or alkaloid drugs—may inhibit absorption.
Aspirin/acetominophen—may increase effects.
Antianxiety drugs—may decrease effects.
Sedative medication—may decrease effects.
Vasoconstrictor drugs—may increase effects.

Comments:
▶ One cup of green tea contains about 40 mg of caffeine.

Capsella bursa-pastoris

Shepherd's purse, capsella, caseweed, mother's heart, pick pocket, shovelweed, witches' pouches

Principal reported indication(s):
Bruising (topical)
Menorrhagia
Metrorrhagia
Nose bleed (topical)
Premenstrual syndrome
Wound healing (topical)

Probable effective dosage:
10–15 grams daily in divided doses as tea

Contraindications:
Cardiac arrhythmias
Cardiovascular disorders
Pregnancy
Renal stones
Thyroid disorders

Potential adverse reactions:
Hypotension
Palpitations
Sedation

Potential medication interactions:
Cardiovascular medication—may increase effects.
Antihypertensive drugs—may increase effects.

Comments:
None

Capsicum spp.

Pepper, chili pepper, cayenne, tabasco, paprika, red pepper

Principal reported indication(s):
Muscle strain (topical)
Neuralgia * (topical)
Nausea
Pains (topical)
Post-herpetic neuralgia (topical)
Rheumatic disorders (topical)
Herpes zoster (shingles) ** (topical)

Probable effective dosage:
Cream/ointment: 0.025% to 0.075% applied 3–4 times daily (wash hands after application)

Contraindications:
Children < 2 years
Damaged skin: lacerations, open wound, or rash

Potential adverse reactions:
Allergic reactions
Burning/itching (topically)
Gastrointestinal discomfort (orally)
Sweating/flushing/lacrimation/rhinorrhea

Potential medication interactions:
No significant medication interactions noted

Comments:
None

Cassia spp.

Senna, te de sena, brica, partridge pea

Principal reported indication(s):
Constipation ***
Hemorrhoids

Probable effective dosage:
0.6–2 grams daily as capsule or tea

Contraindications:
Children < 12 years
Intestinal obstruction
Inflammatory bowel disease
Lactation
Pregnancy

Potential adverse reactions:
Dependence (chronic use)
Intestinal cramping (reduce dosage)
Electrolyte disturbance (with chronic use)
Intestinal pigmentation (benign)

Potential medication interactions:
Cardiac medications affected by potassium depletion
Diuretics—may increase potassium depletion.

Comments:
▶ Stimulant laxatives can cause intestinal cramping
when used alone.

Caulophyllum thalictroides

Blue cohosh, beech drops, blueberry root, blue ginseng, papoose root, squaw root, yellow ginseng

Principal reported indication(s):
Amenorrhea
Dysmenorrhea
Rheumatic disorders
Uterine atony

Probable effective dosage:
0.3–1 gram herb as tea daily

Contraindications:
Gastrointestinal disorders
Pregnancy

Potential adverse reactions:
Fetal cardiac failure
Stomach pain

Potential medication interactions:
Antianginal drugs—may decrease effects.
Antihypertensive drugs—may decrease effects.

Comments:
None

Ceanothus spp.

Jersey tea, New Jersey tea, mountain-sweet, red root, walpole tea, wild snowball

Principal reported indication(s):
Bleeding
Inflammation
Splenomegaly
Upper respiratory infection
Venereal disease

Probable effective dosage:
No dosage noted

Contraindications:
Antithrombotic drugs

Potential adverse reactions:
No significant adverse reactions noted

Potential medication interactions:
Antithrombotic drugs—may increase effects.

Comments:
None

Centaurium spp.

Centaury, bitter bloom, bitter clover, bitter herb, canchalagua, centaury gentian, Christ's ladder, "eyebright," feverwort, fitwort, lesser centaury, minor centaury, rosepink, wild succory, *Erythraea centaurium*

Principal reported indication(s):
Anorexia
Dyspepsia

Probable effective dosage:
2 grams herb as tea 2–3 times daily

Contraindications:
Gastric or duodenal ulcers

Potential adverse reactions:
No significant adverse reactions noted

Potential medication interactions:
No significant medication interactions noted

Comments:
None

Centella asiatica

Gotu kola, hydrocotyle, Indian pennywort,
Indian water navel wort, kola, marsh penny,
talepetrako, thick-leaved pennywort, white rot,
Hydrocotyle asiatica

Principal reported indication(s):
Chronic venous insufficiency **
Hepatic disorders *
Hypertension **
Psoriasis * (topical)
Varicosities *
Wound healing

Probable effective dosage:
0.6 grams of herb as tea 3 times daily
30–60 mg of extract 3 times daily
450 mg capsule daily

Contraindications:
Pregnancy

Potential adverse reactions:
Abortion
Dermatitis
Diabetes
Hypercholesterolemia
Sedation
Urticaria

Potential medication interactions:
Diabetic drugs—may decrease effects.
Hypercholesterol drugs—may decrease effects.
Sedative drugs—may increase effects.

Comments:
▶ *Centella asiatica* should not be confused with
Cola spp.

Cetraria islandica

Iceland moss, consumption moss, fucus, Iceland lichen, muscus

Principal reported indication(s):
Anorexia
Bronchitis/laryngitis **
Dyspepsia/nausea
Mucous membrane irritation
Stomatitis/pharyngitis

Probable effective dosage:
4–6 grams daily

Contraindications:
Gastric/duodenal ulcers
Lactation

Potential adverse reactions:
Gastrointestinal irritation

Potential medication interactions:
No significant medication interactions noted

Comments:
None

*C*helidonium majus

Celandine, felonwort, garden celandine, greater celandine, rock poppy, swallow wort, tetterwort, wart wort

Principal reported indication(s):
Biliary spasm
Cancer
Gastrointestinal spasm
Hepatic disorders

Probable effective dosage:
2–5 grams herb as tea daily

Contraindications:
Children
Lactation
Pregnancy
Use > 2 weeks

Potential adverse reactions:
Dermatitis
Dizziness
Fatigue
Hepatotoxicity
Hypotension
Insomnia
Nausea
Sedation
Toxic reactions have occurred

Potential medication interactions:
Cardiac drugs—may cause arrhythmia.
Diabetic drugs—may decrease effects.
Morphine derivatives—may decrease effects.

Comments:
▶ *Chelidonium majus* has significant toxic potential and is not recommended.

*C*ichorium intybus

Chicory, blue sailors, hendibeh, succory, wild chicory

Principal reported indication(s):
Anorexia
Constipation
Dyspepsia

Probable effective dosage:
3 grams herb daily in divided doses.

Contraindications:
Cardiac arrhythmias
Pregnancy

Potential adverse reactions:
Allergic reaction

Potential medication interactions:
Antiarrhythmic drugs—may decrease effects.

Comments:
None

*C*imicifuga racemosa

Black cohosh, baneberry, black snake root, bugbane, bugwort, rattle root, rattlewood, squawroot

Principal reported indication(s):
Climacteric symptoms ***
Premenstrual syndrome
Dysmenorrhea

Probable effective dosage:
0.3–2 grams as tea 3 times daily

Contraindications:
Lactation
Pregnancy

Potential adverse reactions:
Abortion (large doses)
Dyspepsia/nausea
Toxicity in large doses can cause dizziness, CNS and
   visual disturbances, lowered pulse rate, and
   perspiration.

Potential medication interactions:
Antihypertensive drugs—may increase effects.

Comments:
None

*C*innamomum camphora

Cinnamon, camphor, cassia, Ceylon cinnamon, Chinese cinnamon, false cinnamon, Panang cinnamon, Saigon cinnamon

Principal reported indication(s):
Anorexia
Diarrhea
Dyspepsia *
Flatulence *
Gastrointestinal spasm
Gingivitis

Probable effective dosage:
Use in small quantities as a spice
0.5 grams as tea 3 times daily

Contraindications:
Allergy to cinnamon
Gastric or peptic ulcer
Lactation
Pregnancy

Potential adverse reactions:
Allergic reaction
Mucous membrane irritation
Toxic reaction has resulted from ingestion of 2 oz of cinnamon oil.

Potential medication interactions:
No significant medication interactions noted

Comments:
None

*C*itrus aurantium

Bitter orange peel, Seville orange, sour orange, zhi shi

Principal reported indication(s):
Anorexia
Dyspepsia

Probable effective dosage:
4–6 grams per day as tea, before meal

Contraindications:
Children
Lactation
Pregnancy

Potential adverse reactions:
Photosensitization
Toxic reactions have occurred in children.

Potential medication interactions:
No significant medication interactions noted

Comments:
None

Cnicus benedictus

Blessed thistle, cardin, cardo santo, chardon benit, holy thistle, St. Benedict thistle, spotted thistle

Principal reported indication(s):
Anorexia
Dyspepsia

Probable effective dosage:
1.5–3 grams herb as tea daily

Contraindications:
Allergies to members of the Compositae family
Lactation
Pregnancy

Potential adverse reactions:
Allergic reaction
Stomach irritation and vomiting (high doses)

Potential medication interactions:
No significant medication interactions noted

Comments:
◗ Do not confuse with *Silybum marianum* (milk thistle)

*C*ommiphora molmal

Myrrh, myrra, gum myrrh, hirabol, heerabol,
gummi, bal, bol, African myrrh, Somali myrrh,
Arabian myrrh, Yemen myrrh

Principal reported indication(s):
Gingivitis
Stomatitis/pharyngitis

Probable effective dosage:
As tincture in mouth wash or applied to lesions

Contraindications:
Pregnancy

Potential adverse reactions:
Dermatitis

Potential medication interactions:
No significant medication interactions noted

Comments:
None

*C*ommiphora mukul

Gugulipid, guggul, guggal, gum guggal, gum
guggulu, Indian dellium tree

Principal reported indication(s):
Acne
Hypercholesterolemia **
Hypertriglyceridemia **

Probable effective dosage:
500 mg daily

Contraindications:
Pregnancy

Potential adverse reactions:
Dyspepsia/nausea
Headaches

Potential medication interactions:
Propranol—may decrease effects
Diltiazem—may decrease effects
Thyroid drugs—may increase effects

Comments:
None

*C*onvallaria majalis

Lily of the valley, Jacob's ladder, ladder to heaven, lily constancy, male lily, maybells, May lily, muguet, our lady's tea

Principal reported indication(s):
Cardiac arrhythmia
Cardiac insufficiency
Chronic cor pulmonale
Edema

Probable effective dosage:
0.6 grams standardized powder daily

Contraindications:
Cardiac disorders
Lactation
Pregnancy

Potential adverse reactions:
Cardiac arrhythmias
Dermatitis
Dyspepsia/nausea
Headache
Paralysis
Stupor

Potential medication interactions:
Calcium—may increase effects of herb.
Cardiac drugs—may increase effects.
Corticosteroids—may increase effects.
Diuretics—may increase effects.
Laxatives—may increase effects.

Comments:
▶ *Convallaria majalis* has digitalis-like effects and significant toxic potential. It should not be used.

*C*oriandrum sativum

Coriander, Chinese parsley, cilantro, coriander fruit

Principal reported indication(s):
Anorexia
Dyspepsia

Probable effective dosage:
3 grams daily
10–20 drops tincture after meals

Contraindications:
No significant contraindications noted

Potential adverse reactions:
Allergic reaction
Dermatitis

Potential medication interactions:
No significant medication interactions noted

Comments:
None

Cornus florida

Dogwood, American boxwood, American dogwood, box tree, bitter redberry, budwood, cornel, Cornelian tree, false box, green ozier, osier, rose willow, silky cornel, swamp dogwood

Principal reported indication(s):
Constipation
Infection (topical)
Uterine atony

Probable effective dosage:
No dosage noted

Contraindications:
Pregnancy

Potential adverse reactions:
No significant adverse reactions noted

Potential medication interactions:
No significant medication interactions noted

Comments:
◗ *Cornus florida* tincture was used as a substitute for quinine.

*C*rataegus monogyra

Hawthorn, English hawthorn, haw, hawthorn
tops, may, maybush, mayhaw, oneseed,
whitethorn herb

Principal reported indication(s):
Antiarrhythmic
Congestive heart failure ***

Probable effective dosage:
160–900 mg extract 2–3 times daily

Contraindications:
Children < 12 years
Lactation
Pregnancy

Potential adverse reactions:
Agitation
Circulatory disturbances
Dizziness
Dyspepsia/nausea
Headache
Insomnia
Palpitations

Potential medication interactions:
Cardiovascular drugs—may increase effects.
Coronary vasodilators—may increase effects.
Digoxin—may increase effects.
CNS depressants—may increase effects.

Comments:
- Hawthorn leaf with flower extracts is the form most
  typically used and studied.
- *Crataegus* should only be used under the direction of
  a medical professional.

Cucurbita pepo
Pumpkin

Principal reported indication(s):
Benign prostatic hypertrophy ** +/–
Intestinal parasites (requires large doses) *
Irritable bladder

Probable effective dosage:
5–10 grams seeds per day for BPH
20–150 grams seeds 3 times a day for parasites

Contraindications:
No significant contraindications noted

Potential adverse reactions:
No significant adverse reactions noted

Potential medication interactions:
No significant medication interactions noted

Comments:
▶ Other species may have similar effects.
▶ Trials demonstrate improvement of prostate symptoms without decrease in prostrate size.

*C*uminum cyminum
Cumin

Principal reported indication(s):
Flatulence
Intestinal spasm

Probable effective dosage:
200–600 mg daily in divided doses

Contraindications:
No significant contraindications noted

Potential adverse reactions:
Dermatitis
Photosensitivity

Potential medication interactions:
No significant medication interactions noted

Comments:
None

Curcuma longa

Turmeric, curcuma, Indian saffron, Indian valerian, jiang huang, red valerian

Principal reported indication(s):
Cancer prevention *
Cholelithiasis *
Dyspepsia
Inflammation *
Rheumatic disorders *

Probable effective dosage:
1.5–3 grams daily. Should be taken on an empty stomach.

Contraindications:
Antithrombotic therapy
Bile duct obstruction
Gastric or duodenal ulcers
Immunosuppressive therapy
Pregnancy

Potential adverse reactions:
Dermatitis
Dyspepsia/nausea

Potential medication interactions:
Antithrombotic drugs—may increase effects.
Immunosuppressive drugs—may decrease effects.
NSAIDs—may increase risk of bleeding.

Comments:
None

Cymbopogon spp.

Lemongrass, British Indian lemongrass, capim-cidrao, cochin lemongrass, fevergrass, Guatemalan lemongrass, Madagascar lemongrass

Principal reported indication(s):
Dyspepsia/nausea
Insect repellant (topical)
Myalgias (topical)
Restlessness

Probable effective dosage:
1–2 tsp as tea daily

Contraindications:
No significant contraindications noted

Potential adverse reactions:
Allergic reaction

Potential medication interactions:
No significant potential medication interactions.

Comments:
None

*C*ytisus scoparius

Broom, bannal, basam, bizzom, besom, breeam, broom tops, browne, brum, genista, hog wood, Irish tops, Scotch broom

Principal reported indication(s):
Circulatory disorders
Hypertension

Probable effective dosage:
1–2 grams herb as tea 3 times daily

Contraindications:
AV block
Cardiac pacemaker
Hepatic disorders
Hypertension
MAO inhibitors
Pregnancy
Renal disorders
Splenic disorders

Potential adverse reactions:
Abortion (large doses)
Dizziness (large doses)
Headache (large doses)
Insomnia (large doses)
Palpitations (large doses)
Respiratory failure (large doses)
Sweating (large doses)

Potential medication interactions:
Cardiac drugs—may cause arrhythmias.
Hypertensive drugs—may decrease effects.
MAO inhibitors—may cause hypertensive crisis.

Comments:
▶ *Cytisus scoparius* has significant toxic potential and is not recommended.

*E*chinacea spp.

Echinacea, Kansas snakeroot, purple cone flower, snakeroot

Principal reported indication(s):
Cancer adjuvant
Immunostimulation **
Infections * +/−
Upper respiratory infection *** +/−
Wound healing

Probable effective dosage:
250 mg 3 times a day
30–60 drops tincture 3 times daily

Contraindications:
Autoimmune diseases
Pregnancy

Potential adverse reactions:
Allergic reaction
Dyspepsia/nausea
Numbness of mouth and tongue

Potential medication interactions:
Steroid drugs—may decrease effects.
Immunosuppressive drugs—may decrease effects.

Comments:
▶ *Echinacea* probably should not be taken for more than 3 weeks at a time without discontinuing for a week.

Elettaria cardamomum

Cardamom, bai dou kou

Principal reported indication(s):
Anorexia
Bronchitis/cough
Biliary disorders
Dyspepsia
Flatulence
Hepatic disorders
Infection prevention
Stomatitis/pharyngitis
Upper respiratory infection

Probable effective dosage:
1.5 grams seeds daily
1–2 grams tincture daily

Contraindications:
Gallstones

Potential adverse reactions:
Dermatitis

Potential medication interactions:
No significant medication interactions noted

Comments:
None

*E*leuthrococcus senticosus

*E*leuthrococcus senticosus

Siberian ginseng, eluthera, eluthero, touch-me-not, wild pepper, *Acanthopanax senticosus*

Principal reported indication(s):
Blood pressure disorders
Fatigue; mental or physical *
Immunostimulant +/−

Probable effective dosage:
2–3 grams daily as tea or in capsules

Contraindications:
Hypertension

Potential adverse reactions:
Drowsiness
Hypoglycemia
Cardiac arrhythmias

Potential medication interactions:
Digoxin—may increase effects.
Insulin—may increase effects.
Hormone therapy—may increase effects.

Comments:
▶ Actual quantity of herb in remedies may vary significantly.
▶ *Eleutherococcus* should not be used longer than 3 months at a time.

Ephedra spp.

Ephedra, Brigham tea, herbal ecstasy, joint fir, ma-huang, Mormon tea

Principal reported indication(s):

Allergies	Edema
Asthma **	Fatigue; mental or physical *
Bradycardia *	Nasal congestion
Bronchitis	Obesity *

Probable effective dosage:
15–20 mg 3 times daily

Contraindications:

Anorexia	Cardiovascular disorders
Anxiety	Diabetes
Benign prostatic hypertrophy	Hypertension
	Urinary retention

Potential adverse reactions:

Anorexia	Irritability
Anxiety	Nausea
Dizziness	Palpitations
Headache	Psychosis
Hypertension	Tachycardia
Insomnia	

Toxic reactions, including heart failure and death

Potential medication interactions:
Amphetamines—may increase effects.
Caffeine—may increase effects.
Diabetes drugs—may increase effects.
MAO inhibitors—may increase effects.
Theophylline—may increase effects.

Comments:
▶ *Ephedra nevadensis* (American ephedra) does not contain ephedrine. It is safer and less effective.
▶ *Ephedra* should only be used under the direction of a medical professional.

57

*E*quisetum arvense

Horsetail, common horsetail, bottle brush, Dutch rush, field horsetail, paddock pipes, pewter pipes, scouring rush, shave grass, shavetail grass, toad pipe

Principal reported indication(s):
Renal/bladder stones
Urinary tract edema
Wound healing

Probable effective dosage:
6 grams daily with copious fluid
10 mL tincture 3 times daily

Contraindications:
Children
Edema due to cardiac or renal disorders

Potential adverse reactions:
Dermatitis
Thiamine deficiency
Toxicity similar to nicotine toxicity has occurred.

Potential medication interactions:
Diuretics—may increase effects.

Comments:
None

*E*ucalyptus spp.

Eucalyptus, fever tree, gum tree, malee, Tasmanian blue gum

Principal reported indication(s):
Bronchitis/cough
Congestion +/−
Rheumatism (topical)

Probable effective dosage:
4–6 grams daily in divided doses as tea
10–15 mg tincture 2 times daily
Steam inhalation for congestion

Contraindications:
Children < 12 years
Cholecystitis
Gastrointestinal inflammation
Hepatic disorders

Potential adverse reactions:
Dyspepsia/nausea
Toxic effects including delirium, cyanosis and seizures
    have occurred from ingestion of eucalyptus oil.

Potential medication interactions:
Oral drugs—may decrease effects.

Comments:
None

*E*upatorium perfoliatum

Boneset, agueweed, crosswort, feverwort,
Indian sage, richweed, sweating plant, teasel,
thoroughwort, vegetable antimony

Principal reported indication(s):
Constipation
Edema
Fever
Inflammation

Probable effective dosage:
2–6 tsp in tea daily

Contraindications:
Allergic reaction to Compositae family

Potential adverse reactions:
Allergic reaction
Diarrhea (large doses)
Hepatotoxicity
Vomiting

Potential medication interactions:
No significant medication interactions noted

Comments:
None

Euphrasia spp.

Eyebright, euphrasia, meadow eyebright, red eyebright

Principal reported indication(s):
Conjunctivitis (topical)
Sinusitis

Probable effective dosage:
Gauze soaked in tea and applied to eye several times a day
No internal dosage noted

Contraindications:
No significant contraindications noted

Potential adverse reactions:
Confusion
Congestion
Headache
Inflammation of the eye (topical)
Photophobia (topical)
Sneezing
Weakness

Potential medication interactions:
No significant medication interactions noted

Comments:
▶ No human studies have demonstrated effectiveness of *Euphrasia spp.*
▶ A nonsterile solution could be a source of eye infection.
▶ Use of *Euphrasia spp.* is not recommended.

Filipendula ulmaria

Meadowsweet, bridewort, dolloff, dropwort, gravel root, meadwort, mede-sweet, queen-of-the-meadow, spirea, *Spiraea ulmaria*

Principal reported indication(s):
Anorexia
Bronchitis/cough
Edema
Fever
Rheumatic disorders
Upper respiratory infection

Probable effective dosage:
2.5–3.5 grams flower 3–4 times daily
4–5 grams herb as tea 3–4 times daily
2–4 mL tincture 3 times daily

Contraindications:
Aspirin sensitivity
Asthma—use cautiously

Potential adverse reactions:
Allergic reaction
Bronchospasm
Dyspepsia/nausea

Potential medication interactions:
No significant medication interactions noted

Comments:
▶ *Filipendula* was one of the sacred Druidic herbs.
▶ *Filipendula* was used as the source of salicylates for the development of aspirin in the late 1800s.

*F*oeniculum vulgare

Fennel, carosella, common fennel, finocchio, Florence fennel, garden fennel, sweet fennel, wild fennel, *Anethum foeniculum*

Principal reported indication(s):
Bronchitis/cough
Dyspepsia
Galactagogue
Intestinal spasm

Probable effective dosage:
5–7 grams of crushed seed daily
0.1–0.6 mL oil daily

Contraindications:
Children < 6 years
Pregnancy

Potential adverse reactions:
Allergic reaction
Photodermatitis
Toxicity, including seizures and hallucinations, has occurred with use of essential oil.

Potential medication interactions:
Ciprofloxacin—may decrease effect.

Comments:
‣ In the wild, *Foeniculum* has been confused with hemlock, a very poisonous herb.

Fuycus vesiculosus

Bladderwrack, black tang, bladder focus, cutweed, focus, kelpware, quercus marina, sea oak, sea wrack, *Ascophyllum nodosum*

Principal reported indication(s):
Hypothyroid
Obesity

Probable effective dosage:
5–10 grams of herb as tea 3 times daily

Contraindications:
Antithrombotic drugs
Cancer
Cardiac disorders
Diabetes
Hepatic disorders
Renal disorders
Thyroid disorders

Potential adverse reactions:
Hyperglycemia
Hyperthyroid (large doses)
Nephrotoxicity
Increased thirst
Increased urination

Potential medication interactions:
Antithrombotic drugs—may increase effects.
Diabetic drugs—may decrease effects.
Iron—may decrease absorption.
Thyroid drugs—may increase effects.

Comments:
None

Galega officinalis

Goat's rue, European goat's rue, French honey
suckle, French lilac, Italian fitch

Principal reported indication(s):
Diabetes
Edema
Galactagogue

Probable effective dosage:
2 grams herb as tea daily

Contraindications:
No significant contraindications noted

Potential adverse reactions:
Toxic reaction has occurred in animals (large doses)

Potential medication interactions:
Diabetic drugs—may increase effects.

Comments:
None

*G**alium odoratum*

Woodruff, master of the woods, sweet woodruff, woodwort

Principal reported indication(s):
Bronchitis/cough
Constipation
Dermatitis (topical)
Hemorrhoids (topical)
Varicosities (topical)
Wound healing (topical)

Probable effective dosage:
2 grams as tea daily

Contraindications:
No significant contraindications noted

Potential adverse reactions:
Headache
Hepatotoxicity (chronic use)
Stupor (large doses)

Potential medication interactions:
No significant medication interaction noted

Comments:
None

Gaultheria procumbens

Wintergreen, box berry, Canada tea, checker berry, deer berry, ground berry, hill berry, mountain tea, partridge berry, spice berry, tea berry, wax cluster

Principal reported indication(s):
Myalgias (topical)
Neuralgias (topical)
Rheumatic disorders (topical)
Sciatica (topical)

Probable effective dosage:
10–30% topical oil 3–4 times daily

Contraindications:
Antithrombotic drugs
Children
Esophageal reflux

Potential adverse reactions:
Allergic reaction
Gastric irritation (large doses)
Renal inflammation (large doses)
Toxic reactions have occurred with volatile oils, especially in children.

Potential medication interactions:
Antithrombotic drugs—may increase effects.

Comments:
▶ Significant toxicity can result from internal use and is not recommended.

Gentiana lutea

Gentian, bitter root, bitterwort, gall weed,
gentiana, pale gentian, stemless gentian, wild
gentian, yellow gentian

Principal reported indication(s):
Anorexia
Dyspepsia

Probable effective dosage:
1 gram as tea 3 times daily

Contraindications:
Gastric or duodenal ulcer
Hypertension
Pregnancy

Potential adverse reactions:
Dyspepsia/nausea
Gastric irritation
Headache

Potential medication interactions:
No significant medication interactions noted

Comments:
None

Ginkgo biloba

Ginkgo, kew tree, maidenhair tree

Principal reported indication(s):
Dementia *** +/−
Intermittent claudication ** +/−
Memory loss *
Raynaud's disease
Tinnitus *
Vertigo **

Probable effective dosage:
120–240 mg 2–3 times daily

Contraindications:
Antithrombotic agents

Potential adverse reactions:
Allergic reaction
Bleeding
Dyspepsia/nausea

Potential medication interactions:
Antithrombotic agents

Comments:
None

*G*lycine spp.

Soy, soya, soybean, soybean curd, lecithin, tofu

Principal reported indication(s):
Cancer prevention
Climacteric symptoms *
Hypercholesterolemia *** +/−

Probable effective dosage:
3.5 grams of soy products daily

Contraindications:
No significant contraindications noted

Potential adverse reactions:
Allergic reaction

Potential medication interactions:
No significant medication interactions noted

Comments:
None

Glycyrrhiza glabra

Licorice, Chinese licorice, Persian licorice,
Russian licorice, Spanish licorice, sweet root

Principal reported indication(s):
Cough
Gastritis
Seborrhea
Peptic or duodenal ulcer **
Stomatitis

Probable effective dosage:
2–4 380 mg deglycyrrhizanated licorice (DGL) tablets
  before meals.
1–4 grams of tea or root 3 times daily

Contraindications:
Heart disease
Hypertension
Hypokalemia
Liver disorders
Renal disorders

Potential adverse reactions:
Edema
Hypertension
Pseudoaldosteronism (in chronic high doses)

Potential medication interactions:
Digoxin—with hypokalemia
Diuretics—with hypokalemia

Comments:
▶ DGL has not demonstrated any of the contraindications, potential adverse reactions, or potential
  medication interactions of regular licorice.
▶ Most licorice candy in the U.S. contains anise
  flavoring rather than licorice.

*H*amamelis virginiana

Witch hazel, hamamelis, snapping hazel
spotted alder, tobacco wood, winterbloom

Principal reported indication(s):
Dermatitis (topical)
Eczema (topical)
Hemorrhoids (topical)
Varicose veins (topical)
Wound healing (topical)

Probable effective dosage:
Applied topically as aqueous distillate, ointment or gel
  1–3 times daily

Contraindications:
Internal use

Potential adverse reactions:
Dermatitis
Dyspepsia/nausea/vomiting (internal)
Hepatotoxicity (internal)

Potential medication interactions:
No significant medication interactions noted with topical use.

Comments:
None

*H*arpagophytum procumbens
Devil's claw, grapple plant, wood spider

Principal reported indication(s):
Anorexia
Dyspepsia
Edema
Rheumatic disorders

Probable effective dosage:
1.5 grams as tea daily for anorexia
4.5 grams as tea daily for other uses

Contraindications:
Gastric or duodenal ulcers
Biliary stones
Pregnancy

Potential adverse reactions:
Diarrhea
Headache

Potential medication interactions:
Antithrombotic drugs—may increase effects.

Comments:
None

*H*edera helix
Ivy, English ivy, gum ivy, true ivy, woodbine

Principal reported indication(s):
Bronchitis/cough

Probable effective dosage:
0.3–0.8 grams as tea up to 3 times daily

Contraindications:
No significant contraindications noted

Potential adverse reactions:
Dermatitis

Potential medication interactions:
No significant medication interactions noted

Comments:
None

Humulus lupulus

Hops, common hops, European hops, lupulin

Principal reported indication(s):
Anxiety
Gastric atony
Insomnia ** (in combination with *Valeriana*)

Probable effective dosage:
1–2 grams as tea daily
2.5 mL tincture daily

Contraindications:
Driving or operating machinery

Potential adverse reactions:
Allergic reaction
Bronchial irritation
Dermatitis
Sedation

Potential medication interactions:
Sedatives—may increase effects.
Phenothiazine drugs—may increase effects.

Comments:
None

*H*ydrastis canadensis

Goldenseal, eye balm, Indian paint, jaundice root, orange root

Principal reported indication(s):
Bacterial infection
Diarrhea *
Trachoma

Probable effective dosage:
500–1000 mg 3 times daily

Contraindications:
G6PD deficiency
Pregnancy

Potential adverse reactions:
Bitter taste
Toxic reaction in large doses may cause nausea, vomiting, hypertension, convulsions, and respiratory failure.

Potential medication interactions:
Heparin—may increase effects.

Comments:
◗ *Hydrastis canadensis* is rapidly disappearing in the wild. Other berberine containing plants (barberry, Oregon grape root) should be used in place of this herb.
◗ *Hydrastis canadensis* does ***not*** mask illegal drugs in drug testing.

*H*ypericum perforatum

St. John's wort, amber, goatweed, Klamath weed

Principal reported indication(s):
Anxiety *
Bacterial infection
Depression *** +/–
Viral infection
Wound healing *

Probable effective dosage:
300 mg 3 times daily
Should be taken for at least 4–6 weeks for depression.

Contraindications:
Antidepressant medication
Attempting fertility
Pregnancy
Lactation

Potential adverse reactions:
Dyspepsia/nausea
Fatigue
Photosensitivity
Restlessness

Potential medication interactions:
Antidepressants—may increase effects.
Barbiturates—may increase effects.
Cyclosporin—may decrease effects.
Cytochrome P450 medications—may decrease effects.
Hormones—may decrease effects.
Photosensitizing medications—may increase effects.

Comments:
▶ *Hypericum perforatum* has been shown in human
studies to be effective in mild to moderate depression.
Recent studies have not shown efficacy in moderate
to severe depression.

Ilex paraguariensis

Maté, Jesuit's tea, kali chaye, Paraguay tea, yerba maté

Principal reported indication(s):
Edema
Fatigue (mental and physical)
Headache
Obesity

Probable effective dosage:
2–4 grams as tea 1–3 times daily

Contraindications:
Anxiety
Cardiac arrhythmias
Children
Gastric or duodenal ulcers

Potential adverse reactions:
Anxiety
Hepatotoxicity (chronic use in large doses)
Insomnia
Palpitations
Potential carcinogen
Withdrawal syndrome; headache

Potential medication interactions:
Antianxiety drugs—may decrease effects.
Amphetamine—may increase effects.
Sedatives—may decrease effects.
Theophylline—may increase effects.

Comments:
▶ *Ilex paraguariensis* contains large amounts of caffeine-like substances.

Ilex spp.

Holly, Christ thorn, holm, holme chase, holy tree, hulm, hulver bush, hulver tree

Principal reported indication(s):
Bronchitis/cough
Dyspepsia/nausea
Edema
Jaundice

Probable effective dosage:
4 grams of tea daily

Contraindications:
No significant contraindications noted

Potential adverse reactions:
Dyspepsia/nausea
Toxic reaction (large doses)

Potential medication interactions:
No significant medication interactions noted

Comments:
None

*I*nula helenium

Elecampane, alant, aunee, elfdoc, elfwort, horse elder, horse heal, scabwort, starwort, wild sunflower, yellow starwort, *Helenium grandiflorum, Aster officinalis, Aster helenium*

Principal reported indication(s):
Bronchitis/cough
Parasitic infection
Upper respiratory infection

Probable effective dosage:
1 gram herb as tea 2–4 times daily

Contraindications:
Allergy to Compositae family
Lactation
Pregnancy

Potential adverse reactions:
Allergic dermatitis
Mucous membrane irritation
Toxic reactions including vomiting, spasm, and paralysis have occurred with large doses.

Potential medication interactions:
No significant medication interactions noted

Comments:
None

*I*ris spp.

Iris, black flag, blue flag, daggers, dragon flower, fliggers, flaggon, flag lily, Florentine orris, gladyne, Jacob's sword, liver lily, myrtle flower, orris root, poison flag, segg, sheggs, snake lily, sweet flag, wild iris, yellow flag, yellow lily

Principal reported indication(s):
Biliary disorders
Bronchitis/cough
Constipation
Dermatitis (topical)
Dyspepsia/nausea

Probable effective dosage:
No specific dosage noted

Contraindications:
Gastric or duodenal ulcers
Infectious gastrointestinal disorders
Inflammatory gastrointestinal disorders
Pregnancy

Potential adverse reactions:
Abdominal pain
Dermatitis (topical)
Bloody diarrhea
Mucous membrane irritation
Vomiting

Potential medication interactions:
No significant medication interactions noted

Comments:
▶ *Iris spp.* has significant toxic potential. Its use is not recommended.

*J*uglans spp.

Walnut, Caucasian walnut, English walnut, Persian walnut

Principal reported indication(s):
Dermatitis (topical)
Hypercholesterolemia
Hyperhidrosis

Probable effective dosage:
1.5 grams of herb as tea daily
8–10 walnuts daily for cholesterol

Contraindications:
No significant contraindications noted

Potential adverse reactions:
Potential carcinogen (internal)
Skin discoloration (topical)

Potential medication interactions:
No significant medication interactions noted

Comments:
None

Juniperus spp.

Juniper, cedar, cedron, sabina

Principal reported indication(s):
Dyspepsia/nausea
Edema
Hyperglycemia
Inflammation
Rheumatic disorders
Urinary tract infection
Upper respiratory infection
Wound healing

Probable effective dosage:
1–2 grams of crushed berries or herb as tea 3–4 times
daily

Contraindications:
Inflammatory gastrointestinal disorders
Lactation
Pregnancy
Renal disorders

Potential adverse reactions:
Allergic reaction
Dermatitis
Gastrointestinal irritation
Renal irritation

Potential medication interactions:
Diuretics—may increase effects.
Diabetic drugs—may increase effects.

Comments:
▶ *Juniperus* is a flavoring agent used in gin.
▶ *Juniperus* should not be used longer than 4 weeks.

Krameria spp.

Rhatany, mapato, Peruvian rhatany, pumacuchu, red rhatany, rhatnhia

Principal reported indication(s):
Diarrhea
Hemorrhoids (topical)
Inflammation (topical)
Stomatitis/pharyngitis (mouthwash)

Probable effective dosage:
Tincture painted on affected area 2–3 times daily
1 gram as tea; rinse or gargle 2–3 times daily
No oral dosage noted

Contraindications:
Use > 2 weeks

Potential adverse reactions:
Allergic dermatitis
Dyspepsia/nausea (internal)
Hepatotoxicity (internal)

Potential medication interactions:
No significant medication interactions noted

Comments:
◗ Internal usage can cause gastrointestinal upset and hepatotoxicity.
◗ Internal usage is not recommended.

_L_ _arrea tridentata_

Chaparral, creosote bush, gobernadora, greasewood, hediondilla

Principal reported indication(s):
Cancer +/−
Dermatitis (topical)
Rheumatic disorders
Upper respiratory infection

Probable effective dosage:
Salve 2–3 times daily
Larrea should not be taken internally.

Contraindications:
Larrea has been associated with at least four cases of hepatic toxicity or failure. It should not be taken internally.

Potential adverse reactions:
Contact dermatitis
Hepatic toxicity and failure (internal use)

Potential medication interactions:
No significant medication interactions noted

Comments:
▶ _Larrea_ has been shown to be a potential carcinogen. No evidence of anticancer activity has been demonstrated in humans.
▶ _Larrea_ should not be used internally.

L*aurus nobilis*

Bay laurel, bay, bay leaf, bay tree, daphne, Grecian laurel, laurel, Mediterranean bay, noble laurel, Roman laurel, sweet bay, true bay, *Umbellularia californica*

Principal reported indication(s):
Diabetes
Flatulence
Rheumatic disorders (topical)
Skin stimulant (topical)

Probable effective dosage:
As seasoning; leaves should not be ingested.
Essential oil in ointment or soap (topical)

Contraindications:
No significant contraindications noted

Potential adverse reactions:
Asthma
Dermatitis (topical)
Gastrointestinal trauma from leaves

Potential medication interactions:
Diabetic drugs—may increase effects.

Comments:
▶ *Laurus nobilis* can be used topically or as a seasoning; the leaves should not be taken internally.

*L*avandula spp.

Lavender, aspic, English lavender, French lavender, Spanish lavender, spike lavender, true lavender

Principal reported indication(s):
Anorexia
Anxiety *
Cholestasis
Dyspepsia
Fatigue *
Insomnia *

Probable effective dosage:
2–4 grams as tea 3 times daily
1–2 drops essential oil

Contraindications:
No significant contraindications noted

Potential adverse reactions:
Allergic reaction
Dyspepsia/nausea
Respiratory depression (large doses)

Potential medication interactions:
Sedatives—may increase effects.

Comments:
None

Leonurus cardiaca

Motherwort, I-mu-ts'ao, lion's ear, lion's tail, lion's tart, thro-wort

Principal reported indication(s):
Cardiac failure
Dysmenorrhea
Palpitations
Uterine atony

Probable effective dosage:
4.5 grams of herb as tea 3 times daily

Contraindications:
Lactation
Pregnancy

Potential adverse reactions:
Allergic reaction
Increased bleeding time
Diarrhea (large doses)
Dyspepsia/nausea (large doses)
Photosensitivity (large doses)
Uterine bleeding (large doses)

Potential medication interactions:
Antithrombotic drugs—may increase effects.
Cardiac drugs—may increase effects.

Comments:
None

*L*inum usitatissimum
Flax, linseed, lint bells

Principal reported indication(s):
Constipation
Dermatitis (topical)
Hypercholesterolemia **

Probable effective dosage:
1 tsp whole seed (not ground) in liquid 2–3 times daily

Contraindications:
Esophageal stricture
Gastrointestinal obstruction
Inflammatory bowel disease

Potential adverse reactions:
Allergic reaction
Dyspepsia/nausea
Intestinal obstruction (large doses)

Potential medication interactions:
Laxatives—may increase effects.
Oral drugs—may delay absorption.

Comments:
None

Lobelia inflata

Lobelia, asthma weed, bladder pod, emetic
herb, gag root, Indian tobacco, puke weed,
vomit root, vomitwort, wild tobacco

Principal reported indication(s):
Asthma
Bronchitis/cough
Myalgias (topical)
Smoking cessation * +/−

Probable effective dosage:
100 mg leaf 3–4 times daily
0.6–2 mL tincture 2–3 times daily

Contraindications:
Cardiac disorders
Infectious gastrointestinal disorders
Inflammatory gastrointestinal disorders
Lactation
Pregnancy

Potential adverse reactions:
Diarrhea
Dizziness
Nausea/vomiting
Tremors
Toxic reactions including death have occurred with large
  doses.

Potential medication interactions:
Cardiac drugs—may decrease effects.

Comments:
▶ No efficacy has been demonstrated in humans for
  smoking cessation.
▶ Breakdown products of lobelia are similar to tobacco.
▶ *Lobelia* has significant toxic potential; internal use is
  not recommended.

Marrubium vulgare

Horehound, common horehound, hoarhound, white hoarhound

Principal reported indication(s):
Anorexia
Cough
Dyspepsia
Fever

Probable effective dosage:
1–2 grams as tea 3 times daily
7.5 mL tincture 3 times daily

Contraindications:
Cardiac arrhythmias
Diabetes
Lactation
Pregnancy

Potential adverse reactions:
Cardiac arrhythmias (large doses)
Diarrhea
Hypoglycemia

Potential medication interactions:
Antiarrhythmic drugs—may decrease effects.
Diabetic drugs—may increase effects.

Comments:
None

Matricaria recutita

Chamomile, German chamomile, Hungarian chamomile, true chamomile, wild chamomile, *Chamomilla recutita, Matricaria chamomilla*

Principal reported indication(s):
Dermatitis (topical)
Inflammatory bowel disease
Insomnia
Intestinal spasm (colic)
Stomatitis/pharyngitis
Upper respiratory infection

Probable effective dosage:
1–3 grams as tea 3–4 times daily
15 mL tincture 3–4 times daily

Contraindications:
Allergy to plants in the Compositae family
Pregnancy

Potential adverse reactions:
Allergic reaction

Potential medication interactions:
Alcohol—may increase effects.
Antithrombotic agents (anticoagulants, antiplatelets, aspirin)—may increase effects.
Benzodiazepines—may increase effects.
Sedatives—may increase effects.

Comments:
None

Medicago sativa

Alfalfa, buffalo herb, Lucerne, purple medic, purple medick, purple medical

Principal reported indication(s):
Diabetes
Fungal infection
Galactagogue
Hypercholesterolemia *
Metrorrhagia

Probable effective dosage:
5–10 grams as tea 3 times daily

Contraindications:
No significant contraindications noted

Potential adverse reactions:
Photosensitivity
Seeds (not leaves or stems) have caused at least one case of pancytopenia, and at least one case of reactivation of lupus

Potential medication interactions:
Antithrombotic drugs—may increase effects (large doses).
Diabetic drugs—may increase effects.
Hormone drugs—may decrease effects (large doses).

Comments:
▶ Adulterants in standard preparations have caused *Listeria* infection.

*M*elaleuca alternifolia

Tea tree oil, Australian tea tree oil

Principal reported indication(s):
Infection (topical)
Fungal infections (topical)
Onychomycosis (topical)
Tinia pedis ** (topical)
Upper respiratory infection (inhaled vapors)
Vaginitis (topical)
Wound healing (topical)

Probable effective dosage:
40% concentration for douche 2 times daily
70–100% concentration topically 2 times daily
Melaleuca should not be taken internally.

Contraindications:
No significant contraindications noted for topical use

Potential adverse reactions:
CNS depression (internal use)
Dermatitis (topical)
Dyspepsia/nausea (internal use)

Potential medication interactions:
No significant medication interactions noted

Comments:
▶ *Melaleuca* should not be taken internally.

Melissa officinalis
Lemon balm, balm, sweet balm

Principal reported indication(s):
Anxiety
Dyspepsia/nausea
Graves' disease
Herpetic lesions (topical) *
Insomnia

Probable effective dosage:
1.5–4.5 grams of herb as tea 3–4 times daily
Topical ointment 3–4 times daily

Contraindications:
No significant contraindications noted

Potential adverse reactions:
No significant adverse reactions noted

Potential medication interactions:
No significant medication interactions noted

Comments:
None

_M_entha arvensis

Mint oil, corn mint oil, field mint oil, Japanese mint oil, marsh mint oil

Principal reported indication(s):
Cholestasis
Dyspepsia/nausea
Irritable bowel syndrome
Myalgias (topical)

Probable effective dosage:
3–4 drops of oil in hot water 2–3 times daily
3–4 drops topically as liniment

Contraindications:
Children
Cholecystitis
Hepatic disorders

Potential adverse reactions:
Bronchospasm (inhalation)
Dermatitis
Dyspepsia/nausea

Potential medication interactions:
No significant medication interactions noted

Comments:
None

*M*entha piperita

Peppermint, brandy mint, lamb mint

Principal reported indication(s):
Biliary disorders
Bronchitis/cough
Dyspepsia **
Intestinal spasm **
Irritable bowel syndrome **
Headache **

Probable effective dosage:
3–6 grams as tea 2–3 times daily
0.2 mL essential oil in hot water 2–3 times daily
0.6 mL enteric coated tablet for irritable bowel
  syndrome

Contraindications:
Children—menthol can cause choking and syncopal
  reactions.
Cholecystitis
Cholelithiasis
Esophageal reflux/hiatal hernia
Hepatic disorders

Potential adverse reactions:
Bronchospasm
Dyspepsia/reflux

Potential medication interactions:
Gastric acid blocking drugs—may decrease effects.
Antacids—may decrease effects.

Comments:
▶ Enteric-coated tablets bypass gastric effects to
  help decrease intestinal motility in irritable bowel
  syndrome.

Mentha pulegium

Pennyroyal, American pennyroyal, European pennyroyal, lurk-in-the-ditch, mosquito plant, pudding plant, squaw balm, squaw mint, tick weed, *Hedeoma pulegioides*

Principal reported indication(s):
Abortifacient (see Potential adverse reactions)
Insect repellant (topical)
Menstrual irregularities (see Potential adverse reactions)

Probable effective dosage:
Oil applied topical every few hours
Should not be taken internally.

Contraindications:
Internal use
Lactation
Pregnancy

Potential adverse reactions:
Dermatitis
Toxic effects when taken internally include spontaneous abortion, hepatic failure, nausea, vomiting, delirium, shock, respiratory failure, and death.

Potential medication interactions:
No significant medication interactions noted

Comments:
▶ *Mentha pulegium* should not be taken internally.

M*entha spicata*

Spearmint, curled mint, fish mint, garden mint, green mint, lamb mint, mackeral mint, our lady's mint, sage of Bethlehem, yerba buena

Principal reported indication(s):
Dyspepsia/nausea
Flatulence

Probable effective dosage:
1–4 grams of herb as tea 3–4 times daily

Contraindications:
No significant contraindications noted

Potential adverse reactions:
No significant adverse reactions noted

Potential medication interactions:
No significant medication interactions noted

Comments:
None

M*itchella spp.*

Squaw vine, checker berry, deer berry, one-berry, partridge berry, running box, squaw berry, twin vine, two-eyed berry, winter clover

Principal reported indication(s):
Amenorrhea
Diarrhea
Edema
Galactagogue
Difficult labor

Probable effective dosage:
2–4 grams as tea daily in divided doses
1–2 mL tincture 3 times daily

Contraindications:
Hepatic disorders
Lactation
Pregnancy

Potential adverse reactions:
Gastrointestinal burning
Hepatotoxicity (rare)
Mucous membrane irritation

Potential medication interactions:
No significant medication interactions noted

Comments:
▶ *Mitchella* has significant toxic potential and is not recommended.

*M*onarda spp.

Bergamot, bee balm, blue balm, high balm, horsemint, low balm, monarda, monarda tea, mountain balm, mountain mint, Oswego tea, scarlet monarda, spotted monarda, wild bergamot

Principal reported indication(s):
Dysmenorrhea
Dyspepsia/nausea
Edema
Flatulence
Intestinal spasm
Premenstrual syndrome

Probable effective dosage:
Herb as tea; no dosage noted
2–4 mL of syrup daily

Contraindications:
Pregnancy

Potential adverse reactions:
No significant adverse reactions noted

Potential medication interactions:
No significant medication interactions noted

Comments:
None

*M*yristica fragrans
Nutmeg, mace

Principal reported indication(s):
Diarrhea
Flatulence
Intestinal spasm
Insomnia
Rheumatic disorders (topical)
Stomatitis
Toothache (topical)

Probable effective dosage:
0.3–1 gram as powder up to 3 times daily
2–10 mL tincture daily in divided doses
1–2 drops essential oil on gum for toothache

Contraindications:
Pregnancy (large doses)
Psychiatric disorders (large doses)

Potential adverse reactions:
CNS stimulation (large doses)
Hallucinations (large doses)
Toxic reactions including death have occurred with
    large doses.

Potential medication interactions:
Antidiarrhea drugs—may increase effects.
Psychiatric drugs—may decrease effects.

Comments:
▶ *Myristica* has significant toxic potential and should
  not be used in quantities greater than needed for
  flavoring.

*M*yrtus communis

Myrtle, bridal myrtle, common myrtle, Dutch myrtle, Jew's myrtle, mirth, Roman myrtle

Principal reported indication(s):
Bladder disorders
Bronchitis/cough
Gastrointestinal disorders
Parasitic infections
Wound healing (topical)

Probable effective dosage:
200 mg herb powder daily
1–2 mL essential oil daily
30 grams in cold water as topical wash several times
daily

Contraindications:
Children
Lactation
Pregnancy

Potential adverse reactions:
Allergic reaction
Hypoglycemia
Toxic reactions, including hypotension and respiratory
failure, have occurred.
Topical application in infants and children have caused
respiratory distress and failure.

Potential medication interactions:
Diabetic drugs—may increase effects.

Comments:
▶ Should not be used with infants or children in any
form.

Nepeta cataria

Catnip, cataria, cat mint, cat nep, catrup, cat's play, catwort, field balm, nip

Principal reported indication(s):
Amenorrhea
Anxiety
Edema
Fever
Flatulence
Headache
Insomnia
Upper respiratory infection

Probable effective dosage:
1–2 tsp herb as tea 2–3 times daily
Two 380 mg capsules 3 times daily

Contraindications:
Children
Pregnancy

Potential adverse reactions:
Headache
Malaise
Vomiting (large doses)

Potential medication interactions:
No significant medication interactions noted

Comments:
▶ No studies have demonstrated psychoactive effects in adults. Cats, however, are a different story.

Ocimum basilicum

Basil, common basil, garden basil, holy basil, Saint Joseph's wort, sweet basil

Principal reported indication(s):
Anorexia
Diabetes *
Dyspepsia
Edema
Fever
Flatulence
Rheumatic disorders
Upper respiratory infection
Wound healing (topical)

Probable effective dosage:
2–5 grams powdered herb daily
2–5 grams as tea 1–2 times daily

Contraindications:
Children
Lactation
Pregnancy

Potential adverse reactions:
Potential carcinogen (chronic use)
Hypoglycemia

Potential medication interactions:
Diabetic drugs—may increase effects.

Comments:
▶ Carcinogenic potential precludes chronic use of herb, or use of essential oil.

O enothera spp.

Evening primrose, flor-de-Santa Rita, king-cure-all

Principal reported indication(s):
Attention deficit disorder +/–
Eczema **
Hyperlipidemia
Mastalgia *
Multiple sclerosis +/–
Premenstrual syndrome ***
Rheumatic disorders **

Probable effective dosage:
2–4 grams of oil daily

Contraindications:
Phenothiazine drugs
Pregnancy

Potential adverse reactions:
Dyspepsia/nausea
Headache
Rash

Potential medication interactions:
Phenothiazine drugs—may decrease effects.

Comments:
▶ Efficacy of *Oenothera* is due to content of gamma-linolenic acid (GLA).

*O*riganum vulgare

Oregano, European oregano, mountain mint,
origano, wild marjoram, winter marjoram,
winter sweet

Principal reported indication(s):
Anorexia
Biliary disorders
Bronchitis/cough
Flatulence
Intestinal spasm
Stomatitis/pharyngitis
Upper respiratory infection

Probable effective dosage:
1 tsp herb as tea internally 2–3 times daily
Tea as gargle or topically 2–3 times daily
Two 450 mg capsules internally 1–2 times daily

Contraindications:
Allergic reaction to plants in the mint family
Iron deficiency anemia

Potential adverse reactions:
Allergic reaction
Dyspepsia/nausea (large doses)

Potential medication interactions:
Iron—may decrease absorption.

Comments:
None

*P*anax ginseng

Ginseng, Asian ginseng, Chinese ginseng,
Korean ginseng, Oriental ginseng, red ginseng

Principal reported indication(s):
Central nervous system stimulant *
Diabetes
Fatigue: mental or physical
Tonic for stress **

Probable effective dosage:
1–2 grams daily

Contraindications:
Diabetes: use with caution.
Hypertension

Potential adverse reactions:
Inability to concentrate (chronic large doses)
Hypoglycemia
Nervousness/irritability

Potential medication interactions:
Diabetic drugs—may increase effects.
Warfarin—may decrease effects.

Comments:
▶ Many remedies contain insignificant amounts of ginseng, or use other herbs reputed to have activity like (or even named) "ginseng."

Passiflora spp.

Passionflower, apricot vine, May pea, wild passionflower

Principal reported indication(s):
Anxiety
Gastrointestinal disorders of nervous origin
Insomnia *
Pain

Probable effective dosage:
0.25–1 gram as capsules 3 times daily
2–8 grams herb as tea in divided dose
0.5–2 mL tincture 3 times daily
Daily use for several weeks may be needed for
therapeutic effect.

Contraindications:
Lactation
Pregnancy

Potential adverse reactions:
CNS depression
Vasculitis

Potential medication interactions:
Antidepressant medication—may increase effects.

Comments:
None

*P*ausinystalia yohimbe

Yohimbe, johimbi, yohimbehe, *Corynanthe yohimbi*

Principal reported indication(s):
Erectile dysfunction ** +/−
Hypotension (see Potential adverse reactions) *
Impotence
Xerostomia (decreased salivation)

Probable effective dosage:
5.4 mg 3 times daily for impotence
6 mg 3 times daily for xerostomia

Contraindications:
Cardiac disorders
Children < 18 years
Depression
Female
Gastric or duodenal ulcers
Hepatic disorders
Lactation
Pregnancy
Prostate disorders
Psychiatric disorders
Renal disorders

Potential adverse reactions:
Agitation
Anxiety
Dyspepsia/nausea
Headache
Hypertension
Insomnia
Mania
Renal disorders
Tachycardia

110

Tremor

Toxic reactions, including cardiac failure and death, have occurred.

Potential medication interactions:

Caffeine—may cause hypertension.

Cardiac drugs—may increase or decrease effects.

Ephedra—may cause hypertension.

MAO inhibitors—may increase effects.

Tricyclic antidepressants—may cause severe hypotension.

Comments:

▶ *Pausinystalia yohimbe* should not be used as an herbal remedy. It should only be used under the direction of a medical professional.

Peumus boldus

Boldo, boldine, Boldo-do-Chile

Principal reported indication(s):
Cholestasis
Constipation
Dyspepsia
Intestinal spasm

Probable effective dosage:
3–4.5 grams as tea daily
Oils and distillates should not be used.

Contraindications:
Biliary obstruction
Central nervous system disorders
Hepatic disorders

Potential adverse reactions:
Hallucinations (chronic use)
Motor aphasia (chronic use)
Paralysis (high doses)

Potential medication interactions:
No significant medication interactions noted

Comments:
◗ Oils and distillates contain toxic compounds and
  should not be used.

*P*hytolacca americana

Pokeweed, American nightshade, American spinach, bear's grape, cancer jalap, cancer root, chongras, coakum garget, ink berry, pigeon berry, poke, poke berry, poke salad, red ink plant, scoke, stoke, Virginian poke, *Phytolacca decandra*

Principal reported indication(s):
Constipation
Emetic
Rheumatic disorders

Probable effective dosage:
60–100 mg as emetic
No other dosage noted

Contraindications:
Children
Pregnancy

Potential adverse reactions:
Confusion/stupor
Diarrhea
Dermatitis (topical)
Nausea/Vomiting
Toxic reactions, including convulsions and death, have occurred.

Potential medication interactions:
Depressants—may increase effects.

Comments:
◗ All parts of plant, including raw berries, are toxic except above ground leaves that grow in early spring. Even properly prepared leaves have had toxic effects.
◗ *Phytolacca americana* should not be used.

*P**imenta spp.*

Allspice, clove pepper, Jamaica pepper, pimenta, pimento, West Indian bay, *Eugenia pimenta*

Principal reported indication(s):
Dyspepsia
Flatulence
Intestinal spasm
Myalgias (topical)
Skin irritant (topical)
Toothache (topical)

Probable effective dosage:
1–2 drops essential oil on gum for toothache up to 4 times daily
1–2 tsp powdered herb in water up to 3 times daily
Powdered herb can be mixed with water for paste for topical use.

Contraindications:
Gastrointestinal disorders

Potential adverse reactions:
Dermatitis
Gastroenteritis
Nausea/vomiting
Potential carcinogen
Toxic reactions, including seizures, have occurred with chronic large doses.

Potential medication interactions:
Antithrombotic drugs—may increase effects.
Iron—may decrease absorption.

Comments:
None

Pimpinella anisum

Anise, anise oil, aniseed, sweet cumin, *Anisum spp., Semen anisi*

Principal reported indication(s):
Bronchitis/cough
Dyspepsia
Edema
Flatulence
Intestinal spasm
Lice (topical)
Psoriasis (topical)
Scabies (topical)

Probable effective dosage:
3 grams herb as tea daily in divided doses
0.3 grams essential oil daily

Contraindications:
Pregnancy

Potential adverse reactions:
Allergic reactions including of the skin, respiration, and
  gastrointestinal organs
Dermatitis
Toxic reactions, including nausea, vomiting, seizures,
  and pulmonary edema, have occurred with the use of
  essential oil.

Potential medication interactions:
No significant medication interactions noted

Comments:
None

*P*impinella major

Burnet-saxifrage, pimpernel, piminella, saxifrage

Principal reported indication(s):
Bronchitis/cough
Obstipation
Upper respiratory infection
Varicosities

Probable effective dosage:
6–12 grams herb 3–4 times daily
6–15 mL tincture daily

Contraindications:
No significant contraindications noted

Potential adverse reactions:
Photosensitivity in fair-skinned individuals

Potential medication interactions:
No significant medication interactions noted

Comments:
None

Pinus spp.

Pine dwarf pine, pine oil, pumilio, Scotch fir, Scotch pine, Stockholm tar, Swiss mountain pine, white pine

Principal reported indication(s):
Bronchitis/cough
Fever
Rheumatic disorders (topical)
Stomatitis/pharyngitis
Upper respiratory infection

Probable effective dosage:
2–5 grams as tea 2–3 times daily
Oil should not be used internally. It is used for vapor inhalation or as liniment for topical use.

Contraindications:
Asthma
Children < 12 years

Potential adverse reactions:
Bronchospasm
Dermatitis
Renal toxicity
Toxic reactions, including death, can occur with internal use of essential oil, especially in children.

Potential medication interactions:
No significant medication interactions noted

Comments:
None

*P*iper cubeba

Cubeb, cubeba, cubeb berry, Java pepper, tailed chubebs, tailed pepper, *Cubeba officinalis*

Principal reported indication(s):
Bronchitis/cough
Edema
Flatulence
Urinary tract infection

Probable effective dosage:
2–4 grams of powdered fruit daily
2–4 mL liquid extract daily

Contraindications:
Gastrointestinal disorders
Renal disorders

Potential adverse reactions:
Gastroenteritis
Cystitis

Potential medication interactions:
No specific medication interactions noted

Comments:
None

*P*iper methysticum

Kava kava, awa, kava

Principal reported indication(s):
Anxiety **
Insomnia

Probable effective dosage:
45–70 mg 3 times daily for anxiety
180–210 mg before bedtime for insomnia

Contraindications:
Driving or operating machinery
Endogenous depression
Lactation
Pregnancy

Potential adverse reactions:
Allergic reaction
Dermatitis (long term use)
Diminished alertness and reaction time
Drowsiness
Dyspepsia/nausea

Potential medication interactions:
Alcohol—may increase effects
Sedatives—may increase effects
Benzodiazepines—may increase effects
Beta-blockers—may increase effects
Dopaminergic agents

Comments:
None

*P*lantago spp.

Psyllium, black plantain, blond plantain, broadleaf plantain, common plantain, English plantain, flea seed, great plantain, Indian plantain, lanten, plantain, psyllium seed

Principal reported indication(s):

Anal fissures *

Constipation **

Dermatitis (topical)

Diarrhea

Edema

Hemorrhoids *

Hypercholesterolemia **

Inflammation

Irritable bowel syndrome **

Obesity

Upper respiratory infection

Probable effective dosage:

10–30 grams of seeds daily in divided doses for bowel symptoms

3–6 grams daily for internal uses

Contraindications:

Allergy to *Plantago spp.*

Intestinal infection

Intestinal obstruction

Lactation

Pregnancy

Potential adverse reactions:

Allergic reaction

Abdominal distention

Diarrhea

Flatulence

Gastrointestinal obstruction

Potential medication interactions:

Carbamazepine—may decrease effects.

Diabetic drugs—may increase effects.

Lithium—may decrease effects.

Oral drugs—may decrease absorption.

Comments:

▶ Increasing fluid intake is imperative when using bulk laxatives.

Polygala senega

Senega, milkwort, mountain flax, northern senega, rattlesnake root, seneca, seneca root, seneca snakeroot, senega snakeroot

Principal reported indication(s):
Bronchitis/cough
Upper respiratory infection

Probable effective dosage:
2.5 gram herb as tea 2–3 times daily
2.5–3.5 grams tincture daily

Contraindications:
Fever
Gastritis
Salicylate sensitivity

Potential adverse reactions:
Diarrhea (large doses)
Gastrointestinal irritation (chronic use)
Vomiting (large doses)

Potential medication interactions:
Antithrombotic drugs—may increase effects.
Diabetic drugs—may decrease effects.
Sedatives—may increase effects.

Comments:
None

Polygonum multiflorum

Fo-ti, Chinese cornbind, climbing knotweed, drop berry, flowering knotweed, He-sho-wu, lady's seal, St. Mary's seal, seal root, sealwort, Solomon's seal

Principal reported indication(s):
Constipation
Hypercholesterolemia *

Probable effective dosage:
3–5 grams herb as tea 3 times daily
500 mg tablets 3 times daily

Contraindications:
Diarrhea
Gastric or duodenal ulcer
Inflammatory bowel disorders
Intestinal obstruction
Pregnancy

Potential adverse reactions:

Dermatitis	Hypokalemia
Flushing	Laxative dependency
Gastric irritation	Numbness in extremities
Hepatotoxicity	

Potential medication interactions:
Cardiac drugs—due to potassium loss.
Diuretics—due to potassium loss.

Comments:
◗ Raw and cured *Polygonum* have different chemical compositions and actions. Most adverse effects are associated with the raw root.
◗ Fo-ti-Teng, a commercial preparation, does not contain *Polygonum*.

Populus spp.

Poplar, alamo, aspen, balm of Gilead, balm of Mecca, black aspen, Canadian aspen, European aspen, quaking aspen, tacamahac, trembling aspen, white poplar

Principal reported indication(s):
Bruising/sprains
Fever
Inflammation
Laryngitis (gargle)
Hemorrhoids
Rheumatic disorders

Probable effective dosage:
5–10 grams as tea daily in divided doses

Contraindications:
Antithrombotic drugs
Asthma
Gastric or duodenal ulcers
Renal disorders
Salicylate allergy

Potential adverse reactions:
Allergic reaction
Bleeding
Hepatotoxicity
Tinnitus
Urticaria

Potential medication interactions:
Antithrombotic drugs—may increase effects.
Salicylates—may increase effects.

Comments:
None

Potentilla anserine

Potentilla, cramp weed, goose grass, goose tansy, goosewort, moor grass, prince's feathers, silverweed, trailing tansy, wild agrimony

Principal reported indication(s):
Diarrhea
Dysmenorrhea
Premenstrual syndrome
Stomatitis/pharyngitis

Probable effective dosage:
2 grams herb as tea 2–3 times daily

Contraindications:
No significant contraindications

Potential adverse reactions:
Gastric irritation

Potential medication interactions:
No significant medication interactions noted

Comments:
None

Potentilla erecta

Tormentil, biscuits bloodroot, cinquefoil, earth bank, English sarsaparilla, ewe daisy, five-finger, flesh and blood, sept foil, seven leaves, shepherd's knappary, shepherd's knot, sunkfield, thormantle, *Potentilla tormenta*

Principal reported indication(s):
Diarrhea
Stomatitis/pharyngitis
Wound healing

Probable effective dosage:
4–6 grams herb daily in divided doses
10–20 drops tincture in water as mouth wash

Contraindications:
No significant contraindications noted

Potential adverse reactions:
Dyspepsia
Vomiting

Potential medication interactions:
No significant medication interactions noted

Comments:
None

Primula veris

Cowslip, arthritica, buckles, butter rose, crewel English cowslip, fairy caps, herb perter, key, flower, key of heaven, may flower, our lady's keys, oxlip, paigle, paigle peggle, palsywort, password, peagle(s), petty mulleins, plum rock, primrose, primula, *Primula officinalis*

Principal reported indication(s):
Bronchitis/cough
Upper respiratory infection

Probable effective dosage:
0.5 gram root as tea 2–3 times daily
2–4 grams flower daily in 1–3 doses
1–3 grams of root tincture daily

Contraindications:
Allergy to *Primula veris*

Potential adverse reactions:
Diarrhea
Dyspepsia/nausea

Potential medication interactions:
Diuretics—may increase effects.
Sedatives—may decrease effects.

Comments:
▶ Do not confuse with *Oeonothera spp.* (evening primrose).

Prunella vulgaris

Self heal, all heal, blue curls, brownwort,
brunella, carpenter's herb, consuelda mero,
heart of the earth, hook heal, sicklewort, slough
heel, woundwort

Principal reported indication(s):
Gastroenteritis
Inflammation
Stomatitis/pharyngitis

Probable effective dosage:
1 tsp herb as tea daily

Contraindications:
No significant contraindications noted

Potential adverse reactions:
No significant adverse reactions noted

Potential medication interactions:
No significant medication interactions noted

Comments:
None

Pygeum africanum
Pygeum, African plum tree

Principal reported indication(s):
Benign prostatic hypertrophy ***
Impotence

Probable effective dosage:
100 grams herb daily
100 mg extract daily, or 50 mg 2 times daily

Contraindications:
No significant contraindications noted

Potential adverse reactions:
Gastrointestinal irritation

Potential medication interactions:
No significant medication interactions noted

Comments:
- *Serenoa repens* has been shown to be more effective with fewer side effects than *Pygeum africanum*.
- *Pygeum africanum* decreases symptoms, with little effect on prostate size.

*Q*uercus spp.

Oak, British oak, common oak, encinillo,
Encino, English oak, live oak, oak bark, oak gall,
stone oak, tanner's bark, white oak

Principal reported indication(s):
Bronchitis/cough
Dermatitis (topical)
Diarrhea
Stomatitis/pharyngitis

Probable effective dosage:
One gram herb as tea 3 times daily, or as topical wash

Contraindications:
Cardiac insufficiency
Extensive skin damage
Fever
Infection

Potential adverse reactions:
Allergic reaction
Bowel obstruction
Constipation
Dyspepsia/nausea
Hepatic toxicity (large doses)

Potential medication interactions:
Alkaline or alkaloid drugs—may decrease absorption.

Comments:
None

Rhamnus spp.

Alder, alder buckthorn, black alder, alder dogwood, arrow wood, black dogwood, buckthorn, California buckthorn, cascara sangrada, common buckthorn, dogwood, European black alder, European buckthorn, frangula, highwaythorn, Persian berries, purging buckthorn, ramsthorn, sacred bark, waythorn, *Alnus glutinosa, Frangula alnus*

Principal reported indication(s):
Constipation

Probable effective dosage:
2–5 grams as tea 2 times daily

Contraindications:
Abdominal pain of unknown origin
Cardiac disorders (chronic use)
Children < 12 years
Inflammatory bowel disease
Intestinal infection
Intestinal obstruction
Lactation
Pregnancy

Potential adverse reactions:
Abdominal pain/cramping
Diarrhea
Electrolyte loss (chronic use)
Intestinal spasm
Intestinal pigmentation
Laxative dependence (chronic use)
Nausea

Potential medication interactions:

Cardiac drugs—from electrolyte loss with chronic use.

Corticosteroids—increased electrolyte loss with chronic use.

Diuretics—increased electrolyte loss with chronic use.

Laxatives—may increase effects.

Oral medications—may delay absorption.

Comments:

▶ Stimulant laxatives may cause intestinal cramping when used alone.

Rheum spp.

Rhubarb, Chinese rhubarb, Da-Huang, garden rhubarb, Himalayan rhubarb, Indian rhubarb, medicinal rhubarb, Turkey rhubarb, *Rheum rhubarbarum*

Principal reported indication(s):
Constipation
Diarrhea

Probable effective dosage:
1–2 grams herb daily for constipation
100–300 mg herb daily for diarrhea

Contraindications:
Abdominal pain of unknown origin
Children < 12 years
Inflammatory bowel disorders
Intestinal infection
Intestinal obstruction
Pregnancy
Renal stones
Use > 2 weeks

Potential adverse reactions:
Arrhythmias (chronic use)
Accelerated bone loss (chronic use)
Diarrhea (chronic use)
Edema (chronic use)
Electrolyte loss (chronic use)
Intestinal obstruction
Intestinal pigmentation
Intestinal spasm

Potential medication interactions:

Cardiac drugs—may increase potassium loss with chronic use.

Diuretics—may increase potassium loss with chronic use.

Laxatives—may increase effects.

Comments:

▶ Stimulant laxatives may cause intestinal cramping when used alone.

Rhus glabra

Sumac, polecat bush, smooth, sumach, sweet sumach

Principal reported indication(s):
Enuresis
Irritable bowel disease
Urinary incontinence

Probable effective dosage:
1 gram of powdered herb daily

Contraindications:
No significant contraindication noted

Potential adverse reactions:
Dermatitis

Potential medication interactions:
No significant medication interactions noted

Comments:
None

Ricinus communis

Castor bean, African coffee tree, castor oil, Mexico weed, Palma Christi, tangantangan, oil plant, wonder tree

Principal reported indication(s):
Constipation
Inflammatory skin disorders (topical)
Parasitic infection

Probable effective dosage:
15–60 mL castor oil daily
Ground seeds as paste (topical)

Contraindications:
Abdominal pain of unknown origin
Children < 12 years
Inflammatory bowel disorders
Intestinal infection
Intestinal obstruction
Lactation
Pregnancy

Potential adverse reactions:
Allergic reaction
Diarrhea
Electrolyte loss (chronic use)
Gastric irritation (large dose)
Intestinal spasm (large dose)
Nausea/vomiting (large dose)
Toxic reactions, including death have occurred with ingestion of the bean.

Potential medication interactions:
Laxatives—increased effects.

Comments:
▶ Castor beans are extremely poisonous; fatal toxic reactions have occurred. Only the oil should be used internally.

Rosa spp.

Rose, cabbage rose, Damask rose, dog brier fruit, dog rose fruit, French rose, heps, hipberries, hip fruit, hop fruit, hundred-leafed rose, rose hips, wild boar fruit, wild brier berries

Principal reported indication(s):
Anxiety
Inflammation
Stomatitis/pharyngitis (topical)

Probable effective dosage:
1–2 grams herb as tea, up to 3 times daily

Contraindications:
No significant contraindications noted

Potential adverse reactions:
Allergic reaction
Diarrhea

Potential medication interactions:
Iron—may decrease absorption.

Comments:
None

Rosmarinus officinalis

Rosemary, compass plant, compass-weed, garden rosemary, old man, polar plant, incensor

Principal reported indication(s):
Anorexia
Blood pressure abnormalities
Dyspepsia
Flatulence
Insect repellent (topical)
Rheumatic disorders (topical)

Probable effective dosage:
2 grams of herb as tea 3–4 times daily
Oil should not be used internally.

Contraindications:
Pregnancy

Potential adverse reactions:
Allergic reaction
Dermatitis
Gastric irritation (large doses)
Renal toxicity (large doses)
Toxic reactions have occurred with large doses.

Potential medication interactions:
No significant medication interactions noted

Comments:
▶ Oil can cause toxic reactions and should not be used internally.

Rumex spp.

Yellow dock, curled dock, garden dock, narrow dock, sour dock

Principal reported indication(s):
Biliary disorders
Constipation
Sinusitis
Skin irritant (topical)
Upper respiratory infection

Probable effective dosage:
2–4 grams herb as tea 3 times daily
1–2 mL tincture daily

Contraindications:
Diabetes
Gastric or duodenal ulcer
Hepatic disorders
Intestinal obstruction
Pregnancy
Renal disorder

Potential adverse reactions:
Allergic reaction
Dermatitis
Diarrhea (large doses)
Dyspepsia/nausea
Renal disorders (large doses)
Increased urination (large doses)
Toxic reactions including death have occurred with ingestion of large doses.

Potential medication interactions:
No significant medication interactions noted

Comments:
◗ Stimulant laxatives may cause intestinal cramping when used alone.

Ruscus aculeatus

Butcher's broom, box holly, Jew myrtle, knee holly, kneeholm, pettigree, sweet broom

Principal reported indication(s):
Chronic venous insufficiency ** (in combination with hesperin and ascorbic acid)
Hemorrhoids
Varicosities

Probable effective dosage:
7–10 mg daily of total ruscogenin in standardized preparations

Contraindications:
No significant contraindications noted

Potential adverse reactions:
Dyspepsia/nausea

Potential medication interactions:
No significant medication interactions noted

Comments:
None

Ruta spp.

Rue, garden rue, German rue, herb of grace,
herbygrass, raute, ruda, ruta, vinruta

Principal reported indication(s):

Abortifacient

Ear ache (topical)

Intestinal spasm

Menstrual disorders

Muscle spasm

Rheumatic disorders
(topical)

Sprains and bruising
(topical)

Uterine atony

Probable effective dosage:

0.5 gram of herb as tea 1–3 times daily

Contraindications:

Gastric or duodenal ulcer

Hepatic disorders

Inflammatory bowel disorders

Pregnancy

Reflux

Renal disorders

Urinary tract infection

Potential adverse reactions:

Abortion

Depression

Dermatitis

Gastrointestinal
irritation

Hepatotoxicity

Hypotension

Photosensitivity

Renal toxicity

Sleep disorders

Toxic reactions, including death, have occurred with
large doses.

Potential medication interactions:

No significant medication interactions noted

Comments:

▶ *Ruta spp.* has significant toxic potential; internal use
is not recommended.

*S*alix spp.

Willow, black willow, crack willow, purple willow, violet willow, white willow, willow bark, yellow willow

Principal reported indication(s):
Back pain
Fever
Headache
Rheumatic disorders *
Xerostomia *

Probable effective dosage:
1–3 grams dried bark as tea 3 times daily

Contraindications:
Antithrombotic drugs
Lactation
Salicylate allergy

Potential adverse reactions:
Asthma
Bleeding
Dermatitis
Renal toxicity

Potential medication interactions:
Antithrombotic drugs—may increase effects.
Salicylates—may increase effects, though this has not been demonstrated in humans.
Quantity of constituents may vary considerably with *Salix* species.

Comments:
None

Salvia officinalis

Sage, broad-leafed sage, Dalmatian sage,
garden sage, meadow sage, tree sage, true sage

Principal reported indication(s):
Anorexia
Climacteric symptoms *
Hyperhidrosis **
Memory loss
Stomatitis/pharyngitis

Probable effective dosage:
4–6 grams of herb as tea daily in divided doses
2.5–7.5 grams tincture daily in divided doses

Contraindications:
Pregnancy

Potential adverse reactions:
Chelitis/stomatitis
Dermatitis
Toxic reactions, including convulsions, have occurred
with use of essential oils and alcoholic tinctures.

Potential medication interactions:
Seizure drugs—may decrease effects.

Comments:
None

Sambucus spp.

Elder, black elder, boor tree, bountry, common elder, dwarf elder, elderberry, European elder, ellanwood, ellhorn, flor sauco, red elder, sweet elder

Principal reported indication(s):
Bronchitis/cough
Constipation
Edema
Fever
Influenza
Upper respiratory infection

Probable effective dosage:
3–4 grams of flowers as tea 1–3 times daily
Bark, stems, leaves, and raw berries can be toxic

Contraindications:
No significant contraindications noted

Potential adverse reactions:
Diarrhea
Vomiting
Toxic cyanide reactions have occurred from ingestion of small amounts of leaves, stems, and raw berries.

Potential medication interactions:
No significant medication interactions noted

Comments:
◗ Toxic reactions have occurred from even topical application of bark, stems, and raw berries. *Sambucus ebulus* (dwarf elder) is particularly toxic.

*S*anguinaria spp.

Bloodroot, Indian plant, Indian red plant, red root, red puccoon, tetterwort

Principal reported indication(s):
Cancer of skin (topical)
Gingivitis (toothpaste)
Expectorant
Dental plaque (toothpaste)

Probable effective dosage:
Tincture 0.3–2 mL 3 times daily

Contraindications:
Internal use
Pregnancy
Skin injury

Potential adverse reactions:
CNS depression
Cramping
Mucous membrane irritation
Nausea/vomiting

Potential medication interactions:
No significant medication interactions noted

Comments:
◗ *Sanguinaria spp.* has significant toxic potential; it should not be used internally.

Saponaria officinalis

Soapwort, bouncing bet, bruisewort, crow soap, dog cloves, Fuller's herb, latherwort, old maid's pink, soap root, sweet Betty, wild sweet William

Principal reported indication(s):
Bronchitis/cough
Inflammatory skin disorders
Upper respiratory infection

Probable effective dosage:
1–2 grams herb as tea 3–4 times daily

Contraindications:
Chronic use
Gastric or duodenal ulcers

Potential adverse reactions:
Diarrhea
Gastric irritant
Gastric or duodenal ulcers (large doses)
Gastrotoxicity (chronic use)
Hepatotoxicity (large doses)
Renal toxicity (large doses)
Neurotoxicity (large doses)

Potential medication interactions:
No significant medication interactions noted

Comments:
▶ *Saponaria* has significant toxic potential; internal use is not recommended.

Sassafras albidum

Sassafras, ague tree, cinnamon wood,
common sassafras, sassafrax, saxirax,
Sassafras officinale, Sassafras varifolium

Principal reported indication(s):
Fatigue
Inflammatory skin disorders
Insect envenomation
Rheumatic disorders
Urinary tract infection

Probable effective dosage:
Potential cancer risk precludes its use

Contraindications:
All uses. *Sassafras albidum* is banned for use in the U.S.

Potential adverse reactions:
Abortion
Dermatitis
Hallucinations
Potential carcinogen
Toxic reactions including stupor and death have
    occurred.

Potential medication interactions:
Sedatives—may increase effects.

Comments:
◗ *Sassafras albidum* is banned for use in the U.S. even
    as fragrance or flavoring due to potential cancer risk.

Schisandra chinensis

Schisandra, Bac Ngu Vi Tu, Bei Wu Wei Zi, Chosen-Gomischi, five-flavor-fruit, Gomishi, magnolia vine, Matsbouza, Ngu Mei Gee, northern schisandra, Omicha, southern schisandra, western schisandra

Principal reported indication(s):
Anxiety
Fatigue; mental or physical
Hepatitis *
Inflammatory bowel disease
Insomnia

Probable effective dosage:
100 mg extract capsule 2 times daily
1.5–6 gram herb daily as powder, tincture or extract

Contraindications:
Pregnancy

Potential adverse reactions:
Dermatitis
Depression (rare)
Dyspepsia
Urticaria

Potential medication interactions:
Antidepressants—may decrease effects.
Hepatically metabolized drugs—may increase effects.

Comments:
None

Scutellaria spp.

Skullcap, blue pimpernel, helmet flower, hoodwort, mad-dog herb, mad-dog weed, mad weed, Quaker bonnet, Virginia skullcap

Principal reported indication(s):
Anorexia
Anxiety +/−
Inflammation
Intestinal spasm +/−
Stroke

Probable effective dosage:
1–2 grams herb as tea 3 times daily
1–2 mL tincture 3 times daily

Contraindications:
Hepatic disorders

Potential adverse reactions:
Hepatotoxicity
Toxic reactions, including giddiness, confusion, stupor, and seizure-like activity have occurred with high doses.

Potential medication interactions:
No significant medication interactions noted

Comments:
▶ *Scutellaria spp.* commercial preparations have been contaminated with germander and teucrium; this may account for hepatotoxicity and other toxic reactions.

*S*enecio spp.

Ragwort, cocash weed, coughweed, false valerian, female regulator, golden groundsel, golden ragwort, golden senecio, grundy swallow, life root, squaw weed

Principal reported indication(s):
Bleeding
Diabetes
Hypotension
Menorrhagia
Uterine atony

Probable effective dosage:
Should not be used internally.

Contraindications:
Hepatic disorders
Internal use
Lactation
Pregnancy

Potential adverse reactions:
Allergic reaction
Hepatotoxicity
Potential carcinogen

Potential medication interactions:
No significant medication interactions noted

Comments:
▶ *Senecio spp.* have significant toxic potential and should not be used.

*S*erenoa repens

Saw palmetto, American dwarf palm tree, sabal

Principal reported indication(s):
Benign prostatic hypertrophy ***
Irritable bladder

Probable effective dosage:
320 mg daily

Contraindications:
Hormone therapy

Potential adverse reactions:
Dyspepsia/nausea
Headaches

Potential medication interactions:
Hormone therapy—may decrease effects.

Comments:
None

Silybum marianum

Milk thistle, Marian thistle, St. Mary thistle, *Carduus marianum*

Principal reported indication(s):
Cholelithiasis
Dyspepsia
Hepatitis *
Hypercholesterolemia
Inflammatory liver disease *
Psoriasis
Toxic liver disease *

Probable effective dosage:
140 mg 3 times daily

Contraindications:
No significant contraindications noted

Potential adverse reactions:
Allergic reaction (rare)
Laxative effect (rare)

Potential medication interactions:
Butyrophones
Phenothiazines
Phentolamine
Yohimbine

Comments:
None

*S*milax spp.

Sarsaparilla, Ecuadorian sarsaparilla, Honduras sarsaparilla, Jamaican sarsaparilla, Mexican sarsaparilla, Sarsa

Principal reported indication(s):
Dermatitis
Edema
Fever
Psoriasis
Renal disorders
Rheumatic disorders

Probable effective dosage:
1–4 grams herb as tea 3 times daily

Contraindications:
Renal disorders

Potential adverse reactions:
Asthma (from herb dust)
Diarrhea
Gastric irritability
Renal toxicity

Potential medication interactions:
Digoxin—may increase absorption.
Hypnotic drugs—may decrease absorption.
Oral drugs—may increase or decrease absorption.

Comments:
None

*S*olidago virgaurea

Goldenrod, Aaron's rod, Blue mountain tea,
European goldenrod, sweet goldenrod,
woundwort

Principal reported indication(s):
Edema
Inflammation
Intestinal spasm
Renal or bladder stones
Urinary tract infections

Probable effective dosage:
3–5 grams of herbs as tea 2–4 times daily

Contraindications:
Cardiac disorders
Pregnancy
Renal disorders

Potential adverse reactions:
Allergic reaction

Potential medication interactions:
Diuretics—may increase effects.
Cardiovascular drugs—effects of increased diuresis.
Renal drugs—effects of increased diuresis.

Comments:
None

Sorbus aucuparia

Mountain ash, European mountain ash, quickbeam, rowan tree, sorb apple, sorbi, witchen

Principal reported indication(s):
Constipation
Diarrhea
Edema
Gastric or duodenal ulcers
Gout
Hemorrhoids
Renal disorders
Rheumatic disorders

Probable effective dosage:
One dessert-spoon of freshly pressed juice

Contraindications:
No significant contraindications noted

Potential adverse reactions:
Diarrhea (large doses)
Dyspepsia (large doses)
Local irritation
Mucous membrane irritation
Renal toxicity (large doses)

Potential medication interactions:
No significant medication interactions noted

Comments:
▶ *Sorbus aucuparia* has significant potential toxicity in large doses and is not recommended.

*S*tachys officinalis

Betony, bishopswort, hedge nettles, wood betony, *Betonica officinalis*

Principal reported indication(s):
Anxiety
Bronchitis/cough
Diarrhea
Headache
Stomatitis/pharyngitis

Probable effective dosage:
No specific dosage noted

Contraindications:
Pregnancy

Potential adverse reactions:
Gastric irritation
Hepatotoxicity

Potential medication interactions:
Hypertensive drugs—may increase effects.

Comments:
None

*S*tellaria media

Chickweed, adders' tongue, mouse ear, passerina, satin flower, star chickweed, starweed, stitchwort, tongue grass, white birds' eye, winter weed

Principal reported indication(s):
Asthma
Constipation
Dermatitis (topical)
Dyspepsia
Eczema (topical)
Wound healing (topical)

Probable effective dosage:
1–2 tsp herb as tea several times daily

Contraindications:
No significant contraindications noted

Potential adverse reactions:
Paralysis (large doses)

Potential medication interactions:
No significant medication interactions noted

Comments:
None

*S*tevia rebaudiana

Stevia, azucacaa, kaa jhee, Paraguayan sweet herb, sweetleaf, sweet leaf of Paraguay, yerba dulce

Principal reported indication(s):
Constipation
Diabetes
Hypertension
Obesity
Sweetener

Probable effective dosage:
1000 mg daily in divided doses

Contraindications:
Renal disorders

Potential adverse reactions:
No significant adverse reactions noted

Potential medication interactions:
Diabetic drugs—may increase effects.
Hypertensive drugs—may increase effects.

Comments:
▶ *Stevia rebaudiana* has not been approved by numerous international regulatory agencies due to questions about safety. Use cannot be recommended.

Symphytum officinale

Comfrey, ass ear, black root, blackwort, bruisewort, common comfrey gum plant, healing herb, knitback, knitbone, Russian comfrey, salsify, slippery root, wallwort

Principal reported indication(s):
Bruises (topical)
Burns (topical)
Fractures (topical)
Rheumatic diseases * (topical)
Sprains (topical)

Probable effective dosage:
5–20% ointment several times daily. Do not use more than 4–6 weeks per year.
Should not be taken internally.

Contraindications:
Internal use
Lactation
Open wounds
Pregnancy

Potential adverse reactions:
Potential carcinogen
Gastrointestinal toxicity
Hepatotoxicity
Pancreatic toxicity
Renal toxicity

Potential medication interactions:
No significant medication interactions noted

Comments:
▶ *Symphytum officinale* has significant potential toxicity and should not be used internally.

Syzygium aromaticum

Cloves, caryophyllus, Clous de Girolfe, *Eugenia caryophyllata, Caryophyllus aromaticus*

Principal reported indication(s):
Fever
Fungal infection (topical)
Gastric ulcer
Intestinal spasm
Stomatitis/pharyngitis
Tooth pain (topical)

Probable effective dosage:
1–5% clove oil as mouthwash several times daily
120–300 mg several times daily

Contraindications:
Antithrombotic drugs

Potential adverse reactions:
Allergic reaction
Dermatitis (topical)
Hemoptysis (smoked herb)
Mucous membrane irritation (topical)
Pulmonary toxicity (smoked herb)
Toxic reactions including coagulation disorders, depression, and electrolyte disturbances have occurred with the use of essential oil.

Potential medication interactions:
Antithrombotic drugs—may increase effects.

Comments:
▶ Internal use or use of clove cigarettes is not recommended.

Tabebuia spp.

Pau d'Arco, ipe, ipe roxo, ipes, lapacho, lapacho morado, purple lapacho, red lapacho, taheebo, taheebo tea, trumpet bush, *Lapacho colorado*

Principal reported indication(s):
Bacterial infection
Cancer +/−
Dyspepsia
Fungal infection +/−

Probable effective dosage:
1–2 460 mg capsules 2 times daily
15–20 grams bark as tea several times daily

Contraindications:
Antithrombotic drugs
Pregnancy

Potential adverse reactions:
Anemia
Bleeding
Diarrhea
Dizziness
Nausea/vomiting

Potential medication interactions:
Antithrombotic drugs—may increase effects.

Comments:
❯ *Tabebuia spp.* has significant potential toxicity and should not be used.

*T*anacetum parthenium

Feverfew, altamisa, bachelor's buttons, nose
bleed, Santa Maria, wild chamomile, wild
quinine, *Chrysanthemum parthenium*

Principal reported indication(s):
Asthma
Dysmenorrhea
Fever
Inflammation
Migraine headache
Migraine headache prophylaxis ***
Rheumatic disorders

Probable effective dosage:
25 mg freeze-dried extract daily for prophylaxis

Contraindications:
Children < 12 years
Lactation
Pregnancy

Potential adverse reactions:
Allergic reaction
Stomatitis
Withdrawal syndrome (chronic use): pain in muscle,
joints, and tissue

Potential medication interactions:
Antithrombotic drugs—may increase effects.
Nonsteroidal anti-inflammatory drugs—may decrease
effectiveness of *Tanacetem*.

Comments:
▶ Freeze-dried herbs may be only preparations that
are effective for migraine.
▶ *Tanacetum* should not be used for more than
4 months at a time.

*T*anacetum vulgare

Tansy, bitter buttons, buttons, daisy, golden
buttons, hindheal, parsley fern, scented fern,
stinking willie, *Chrysanthemum vulgaris*

Principal reported indication(s):
Abortifacient
Anorexia
Headache
Parasitic infection
Uterine atony

Probable effective dosage:
Dosage not specified
Do not use internally

Contraindications:
Internal use
Lactation
Pregnancy

Potential adverse reactions:
Allergic rhinitis
Dermatitis (topical)
Renal toxicity
Toxic reactions, including renal tumors, arrhythmias,
    and death, have occurred.

Potential medication interactions:
Diabetic drugs—may increase effects.

Comments:
◗ *Tanacetum vulgare* has significant potential toxicity
    and should not be used.

T*araxacum officinale*

Dandelion, blowball, common dandelion, cankerwort, lion's teeth, priest's crown, swine snout, wild endive, *Leontodon taraxacum*

Principal reported indication(s):
Anorexia
Biliary disorders
Dyspepsia
Edema
Hepatic disorders
Urinary tract infection

Probable effective dosage:
3–4 grams as tea 2–3 times daily
5–10 mL tincture 3 times daily

Contraindications:
Biliary obstruction/stone
Intestinal obstruction

Potential adverse reactions:
Allergic reaction
Biliary inflammation
Biliary obstruction
Dermatitis

Potential medication interactions:
Diuretics—may increase effects.

Comments:
None

Thuja occidentalis

Yellow cedar, American arborvitae, arborvitae, eastern arborvitae, eastern white cedar, false white cedar, hackmatack, northern white cedar, swamp cedar, thuga, thuja, tree of life, white cedar

Principal reported indication(s):
Abortifacient
Cancer +/−
Cardiac insufficiency
Fatigue, mental
Herpetic lesions (topical)
Parasitic infection
Upper respiratory infection
Uterine atony

Probable effective dosage:
1 tsp herb as tea 3 times daily
1–2 mL liquid extract 3 times daily

Contraindications:
Gastritis
Gastric ulcer
Pregnancy
Seizure disorders

Potential adverse reactions:
Asthma
CNS stimulation
Flatulence
Gastric irritation
Seizures
Spontaneous abortion
Toxic reactions, including vomiting, diarrhea, hypotension, mucous membrane bleeding, seizures, and death, have resulted from large doses.

Potential medication interactions:

Iron—may decrease absorption.

Sedatives—may decrease effects.

Seizure drugs—may decrease effects.

Stimulants—may increase effects.

Comments:

▶ *Thuja* has significant toxic potential; its use is not recommended.

Thymus vulgaris

Thyme, common thyme, French thyme, garden thyme, red thyme, rubbed thyme, Spanish thyme, timo, white thyme

Principal reported indication(s):
Bronchitis/cough
Gingivitis
Intestinal spasm
Stomatitis/pharyngitis
Upper respiratory infection

Probable effective dosage:
1.5–2 gram herb as tea 2–3 times daily

Contraindications:
Gastritis
Inflammatory bowel disease
Pregnancy

Potential adverse reactions:
Allergic reactions
Toxic effects have occurred with use of essential oil.

Potential medication interactions:
No significant medication interactions noted

Comments:
▶ Toxic effects have occurred with internal use of essential oil and is not recommended.

*T*ilia spp.

Linden, European linden, large-leafed linden, "lime," Linn flowers

Principal reported indication(s):
Anxiety
Bronchitis/cough
Fever
Insomnia

Probable effective dosage:
2 grams herb as tea 1–2 times daily
10 mL tincture 1–2 times daily

Contraindications:
Cardiac disorders

Potential adverse reactions:
Urticaria (topical use)
Cardiac toxicity (chronic use)

Potential medication interactions:
No significant medication interactions noted

Comments:
None

*T*rifolium pratense

Red clover, beebread, cow clover, cowgrass, genistein, meadow clover, pavine clover, purple clover, trefoil, trifolium, wild clover

Principal reported indication(s):
Abdominal cramps
Benign prostatic hypertrophy **
Bronchitis/cough
Cancer prevention
Dyspepsia
Eczema (topical)
Immune-stimulant
Osteoporosis * +/−

Probable effective dosage:
1–2 grams herb as tea 3 times daily
1.5–3 mL tincture 3 times daily

Contraindications:
Antithrombotic drugs

Potential adverse reactions:
Dermatitis

Potential medication interactions:
Antithrombotic drugs—may increase effects.

Comments:
None

*T*rigonella foenum-graecum

Fenugreek, bird's foot, Greek hay seed

Principal reported indication(s):
Anorexia
Dermatitis
Diabetes *
Hypercholesterolemia **

Probable effective dosage:
0.5–2 grams as tea (cold water) 3–4 times daily

Contraindications:
Antithrombotic drugs
Pregnancy

Potential adverse reactions:
Allergic reaction
Bleeding/bruising
Dermatitis
Hypoglycemia

Potential medication interactions:
Antithrombotic drugs—may increase effects.
Diabetes drugs—may increase effects.

Comments:
None

Trillium erectum

Beth root, birth root, coughroot, ground lily, Jew's harp plant, Indian balm, Indian shamrock, lamb's quarters, milk ipecac, Pariswort, purple trillium, rattlesnake root, snakebite, stinking Benjamin, three-leafed nightshade, wake robin

Principal reported indication(s):
Bruises (topical)
Dyspepsia
Menorrhagia
Varicosities (topical)

Probable effective dosage:
2–4 grams herb as tea daily
Topically as poultice

Contraindications:
Cardiac disorders
Lactation
Pregnancy

Potential adverse reactions:
Cardiac toxicity
Gastrointestinal irritation
Vomiting

Potential medication interactions:
Cardiac drugs—may increase or decrease effects.

Comments:
None

Turnera diffusa

Damiana, damiana leaf, herba de la pastora, Mexican damiana, mizibcoc, old woman's broom, "rosemary," *Damiana aphrodisiaca, Turnera aphrodisiaca, Turnera microphylla*

Principal reported indication(s):
Aphrodisiac
Fatigue, mental and physical
Headache

Probable effective dosage:
2–4 grams herb as tea daily
1.5 mL tincture 3 times daily

Contraindications:
Hepatic disorders
Seizure disorders
Urinary disorders

Potential adverse reactions:
Hallucinations
Hepatotoxicity
Seizures
Urethral irritation

Potential medication interactions:
No significant medication interactions noted

Comments:
▶ *Turnera* has significant potential toxicity and should not be used.
▶ Reports of use of smoked *Turnera* as a euphoric or hallucinogen have not been substantiated.

Tussilago farfara

Coltsfoot, ass's foot, British tobacco, bullsfoot, coughwort, flower velure, foal's foot, foalswort, hallfoot, horsefoot, horsehoof, kuandong hua, pas Diane, pas d'Ane, tussilage

Principal reported indication(s):
Asthma
Bronchitis/cough
Dermatitis (topical)

Probable effective dosage:
1.5–2.5 grams herb as tea daily in divided doses
2–8 mL tincture 3 times daily
2 mL liquid extract 3 times daily

Contraindications:
Cardiac disorders
Hepatic disorders
Lactation
Pregnancy

Potential adverse reactions:
Allergic reaction
Anorexia
Potential carcinogen
Diarrhea
Hepatotoxicity
Nausea/Vomiting

Potential medication interactions:
Cardiac drugs—may decrease effects.
Hypertensive drugs—may decrease effects.

Comments:
▶ *Tussilago farfara* has significant toxic potential and should not be used internally.

*U*lmus rubra

Slippery elm, American elm, Indian elm, moose elm, red elm, sweet elm

Principal reported indication(s):
Burns
Bronchitis/cough
Constipation
Dermatitis (topical)
Diarrhea
Gastritis
Gastric and duodenal ulcers
Rheumatic disorders (topical)
Wound healing (topical)

Probable effective dosage:
4 grams herb as tea 3 times daily
5 mL liquid extract 3 times daily
Lozenges for sore throat several times daily

Contraindications:
Pregnancy

Potential adverse reactions:
Allergic reaction
Dermatitis
Spontaneous abortion

Potential medication interactions:
Oral drugs—may decrease absorption.

Comments:
None

Unicaria spp.

Cat's claw, life-giving-vine-of-Peru, samento, una de gato

Principal reported indication(s):
Dyspepsia/nausea
Cancer
Contraceptive
HIV infection
Immune stimulant
Inflammation
Inflammatory bowel disease
Viral disorders

Probable effective dosage:
0.5–1 gram 3 times daily

Contraindications:
Antithrombotic drugs
Children
Immunosuppression
Pregnancy

Potential adverse reactions:
Diarrhea
Hypotension

Potential medication interactions:
Antihypertensive drugs—may increase effects.
Antithrombotic drugs—may increase effects.
Immunosuppressive drugs—may decrease effects.

Comments:
None

*U*rtica spp.

Stinging nettle, common nettle, great stinging nettle, nettle, small nettle

Principal reported indication(s):
Allergic rhinitis **
Benign prostatic hypertrophy **
Bladder irritation
Edema
Renal or bladder stones
Rheumatic disorders
Urinary tract infection

Probable effective dosage:
1–2 grams as tea 2–3 time daily
1–2 freeze-dried capsules every 3–4 hours for allergic rhinitis

Contraindications:
Cardiac failure
Renal failure

Potential adverse reactions:
Dyspepsia/nausea
Topical irritation

Potential medication interactions:
Diclofenac—may increase effects.

Comments:
None

*U*snea spp.

Usnea, beard moss, old man's beard, tree's dandruff, tree moss, woman's long hair

Principal reported indication(s):
Stomatitis/pharyngitis

Probable effective dosage:
100 mg herb in lozenges 3–6 times daily

Contraindications:
No significant contraindications noted

Potential adverse reactions:
No significant adverse reactions noted

Potential medication interactions:
No significant medication interactions noted

Comments:
None

V*accinium macrocarpon*

Cranberry

Principal reported indication(s):
Urinary tract infection
Urinary tract infection: prevention **
Urinary incontinence: deodorizes urine

Probable effective dosage:
3 oz juice daily for prevention of infection
12–32 oz juice daily for treatment of infection

Contraindications:
Lactation
Pregnancy

Potential adverse reactions:
No significant adverse reactions noted

Potential medication interactions:
No significant medication interactions noted

Comments:
None

*V*accinium myrtillus

Bilberry, bog bilberry, European blue
berry, huckleberry, whortle berry,
Myrtillus fructus

Principal reported indication(s):
Diabetic retinopathy +/−
Diarrhea
Stomatitis/pharyngitis
Vision—enhances night vision +/−
Wound healing

Probable effective dosage:
60–160 mg 3 times daily

Contraindications:
Antithrombotic agents

Potential adverse reactions:
No significant adverse reactions noted

Potential medication interactions:
Antithrombotic agents—may increase effects.

Comments:
None

Valeriana spp.

Valerian all-heal, amantilla, garden valerian, heliotrope, Indian valerian, Mexican valerian

Principal reported indication(s):
Anxiety
Dysmenorrhea
Insomnia ***
Irritable bowel disease

Probable effective dosage:
1–2 grams as tea 2–3 times daily or at bedtime
150 mg capsule 2–3 times daily or at bedtime

Contraindications:
Driving or operating machinery
Lactation
Pregnancy

Potential adverse reactions:
Drowsiness
Dyspepsia/nausea

Potential medication interactions:
Alcohol—may increase effects.
Barbiturates—may increase effects.
Benzodiazepines—may increase effects.

Comments:
▶ The herb stinks!

V*eratrum viride*

Hellebore, American veratrum, American
white hellebore, bugbane, devil's bite, earth
gall, false hellebore, green hellebore, green
veratrum, Indian poke, itchweed, tickleweed

Principal reported indication(s):
Hypertension
Tachycardia

Probable effective dosage:
100 mg powdered herb daily

Contraindications:
Internal use
Cardiac disorders
Gastrointestinal disorders
Lactation
Pregnancy

Potential adverse reactions:
Toxic reactions including diarrhea, vomiting, paralysis,
seizures, cardiac arrhythmias, hypotension, and death
have occurred.

Potential medication interactions:
Cardiac drugs—may increase effects.
Hypertensive drugs—may increase effects.

Comments:
◗ *Veratrum viride* has significant toxic potential and
should not be used.

Verbascum spp.

Mullien, blanket lead, bunny ears, candle wick, flannel mullien, large-flowered mullien, Jacob's staff, torch weed, velvet plant

Principal reported indication(s):
Bronchitis/cough
Earache (topical oil)
Upper respiratory infection
Wound healing (topical)

Probable effective dosage:
1.5–2 grams herb as tea 2–3 times daily
20–30 drops tincture several times daily

Contraindications:
No significant contraindications noted

Potential adverse reactions:
Dermatitis
Sedation

Potential medication interactions:
No significant medication interactions noted

Comments:
None

*V*erbena spp.

Vervain, blue vervain, common verbena, common vervain, enchanter's plant, European vervain, herb of grace, herb of the cross, holywort, Juno's tears, pigeon's grass, pigeonweed, simpler's joy, turkey grass

Principal reported indication(s):
Asthma
Bronchitis/cough
Cramps
Insomnia
Pain
Rheumatic disorders
Stomatitis/pharyngitis
Wound healing (topical)

Probable effective dosage:
2–4 grams herb as tea 3 times daily
5–10 mL tincture 3 times daily
2–4 mL liquid extract daily

Contraindications:
Pregnancy
Seizure disorders

Potential adverse reactions:
Dermatitis
Paralysis (large doses)
Seizures (large doses)

Potential medication interactions:
Seizure drugs—may decrease effects.

Comments:
None

Viburnum prunifolium

Black haw, American sloe, European cranberry, crampbark, dog rowan tree, guelder rose, king's crown, high cranberry, may rose, nanny berry, red elder, rose elder, wheep berry, shonny, silver bells, sloe, snowball tree, southern black haw, stag bush, water elder, whitsun bosses

Principal reported indication(s):
Diarrhea
Dysmenorrhea
Edema

Probable effective dosage:
2 tsp bark as tea 3 times daily
3–10 mL tincture 3 times daily

Contraindications:
Pregnancy
Lactation

Potential adverse reactions:
Allergic reaction
Gastrointestinal irritation

Potential medication interactions:
No significant medication interactions noted

Comments:
None

V*inca minor*

Periwinkle, common periwinkle, earlyflowering, evergreen, lesser periwinkle, "myrtle," small periwinkle, "wintergreen"

Principal reported indication(s):
Cancer (in purified, standarized medical preparation)
Circulatory disorders
Fatigue, mental
Memory loss

Probable effective dosage:
1 tsp herb as tea 2–3 times daily

Contraindications:
Cardiac disorders
Constipation
Hypertension

Potential adverse reactions:
Dyspepsia/nausea
Flushing
Hypotension
Hepatotoxicity
Neurotoxicity
Renal toxicity

Potential medication interactions:
Cardiac drugs—may decrease effects.
Hypertensive drugs—may increase effects.
Laxatives—may increase effects.

Comments:
◗ *Vinca minor* has significant toxic potential and should not be used.

V*iscum album*

Mistletoe, American mistletoe, all heal, birdlime mistletoe, devil's fuge, European mistletoe, leimmistel, *Loranthus spp., Phoradendron spp.*

Principal reported indication(s):
Anxiety
Bleeding
Cancer adjuvant +/−
Fatigue, mental
Hypertension/hypotension (dose dependent)
Rheumatic disorders
Uterine atony

Probable effective dosage:
2.5 grams herb as tea 1–2 times daily
0.5 mL tincture 3 times daily

Contraindications:
Internal use
Antithrombotic drugs
Cardiac disorders
Hypertension
Hypotension
Lactation
Seizure disorders
Pregnancy

Potential adverse reactions:
Allergic reaction
Bradycardia
Delirium
Gastrointestinal irritation
Hypertension
Hypotension
Seizures
Toxic reactions, including hypertension, hallucinations, vasoconstriction, cardiac arrest, and death, have occurred.

Potential medication interactions:

Cardiac drugs—may decrease effects.

Hypertensive drugs—may increase or decrease effects.

Immunosuppressive drugs—may decrease effects.

Sedatives—may increase effects.

Comments:

▶ *Viscum album* has significant toxic potential and should not be used.

▶ *Loranthus spp., Phoradendron spp.* (American mistletoe) are considered to have similar constituents and effects.

*V*itex agnus castus

Chaste tree, chasteberry, monk's pepper

Principal reported indication(s):
Premenstrual syndrome
Climacteric symptoms

Probable effective dosage:
0.5–1 gram 3 times daily

Contraindications:
Lactation
Pregnancy

Potential adverse reactions:
Allergic reaction
Dyspepsia/nausea
Menorrhagia
Dermatitis

Potential medication interactions:
Dopaminergic receptor agonists—may decrease effects.

Comments:
None

Vitis vinifera

Grape seed, grape seed extract

Principal reported indication(s):
Antioxidant
Arteriosclerosis
Chronic venous insufficiency **
Inflammation
Varicosities
Wound healing

Probable effective dosage:
50 mg of extract daily as antioxidant
50–100 mg of extract 3 times daily

Contraindications:
No significant contraindications noted

Potential adverse reactions:
No significant potential adverse reactions noted

Potential medication interactions:
No significant potential medication interactions noted

Comments:
None

Zanthoxylum americanum

Prickly ash, angelica tree, northern prickly ash, pepper wood, suterberry, toothache bark, xanthoxylum, yellow wood

Principal reported indication(s):
Circulatory disorders
Cramps
Fever
Hypotension
Inflammation
Rheumatic disorders

Probable effective dosage:
1–3 grams dried bark as tea 3 times daily
2–5 mL tincture 3 times daily
1–3 mL liquid extract 3 times daily

Contraindications:
Gastrointestinal disorders

Potential adverse reactions:
Salivation (large doses)
Hypertension (large doses)

Potential medication interactions:
No significant medication interactions noted

Comments:
None

Zingiber officinale

Ginger, ginger root

Principal reported indication(s):
Dyspepsia
Hyperemesis gravidarum * (see Contraindications)
Inflammation *
Motion sickness **
Nausea ** +/−
Rheumatic disorders *
Vomiting

Probable effective dosage:
0.5–1 gram 3–4 times daily

Contraindications:
Antithrombotic drugs
Pregnancy—large doses may stimulate uterine
    contractions.

Potential adverse reactions:
Cardiac arrhythmias (large doses)
CNS depression (large doses)

Potential medication interactions:
Antithrombotic drugs—may increase effects.

Comments:
None

References

Physicians Desk Reference for Herbal Medicines, Second Edition. Montvale, NJ: Medical Economics Company, 2000.

Blumenthal, M., Goldberg, A., Brinckmann, J. *Herbal Medicine Expanded Commission E Monographs, First Edition.* Newton, MA: Integrative Medicine Communications, 2000.

Griffith, H., Thompson, C. *Healing Herbs: The Essential Guide.* Tucson, AZ: Fisher Books, 2000.

Dermarderosian, A. *A Guide to Popular Natural Products.* St. Louis, MO: Facts and Comparisons, 1999.

Nurse's Handbook of Alternative and Complementary Therapies. Springhouse, PA: Spring House Corporation, 1999.

Jellin, J., Batz, F., Hitchens, K. *Natural Medicine Comprehensive Database, Second Edition.* Stockton, CA: Therapeutic Research Faculty, 1999.

Duke, J.A. *The Green Pharmacy.* Emmaus, PA: Rodale Press, 1997.

Murray, M.T. *The Healing Power of Herbs, Second Edition.* Rocklin, CA: Prima Publishing, 1995.

Moore, M. *Medicinal Plants of the Mountain West, First Edition.* Santa Fe, NM: Museum of New Mexico Press, 1979.

Moore, M. *Medicinal Plants of the Desert and Canyon West.* Santa Fe, NM: Museum of New Mexico Press, 1989.

Moore M. *Medicinal Plants of the Pacific West, First Edition.* Santa Fe, NM: Red Crane Press, 1993.

Tyler, V.E. *The Honest Herbal, Third Edition.* Binghamton, NY: The Haworth Press, 1993.

Weil, A. *Natural Health, Natural Medicine: A Comprehensive Manual for Wellness and Self Care.* Boston, MA: Houghton Mifflin Company, 1990.

G*lossary*

abortifacient: anything that induces or causes an abortion.

adjuvant: something that assists the effect of an intervention.

alopecia: loss of hair.

amenorrhea: absence or suppression of menstruation.

angina: heart pain due to decreased blood flow to the heart.

anorexant: substance that decreases appetite.

anorexia: loss of appetite, inability to eat.

antianginal: drugs used for angina (decreased blood flow to the heart).

anticholinergic: substance that inhibits the release of acetylcholine, and therefore, inhibits the parasympathetic nervous system.

antiseptic: a substance that arrests or prevents the growth of microorganisms.

antithrombotic agents: substances that prevent the clotting of blood, such as aspirin, heparin, or coumadin.

arrhythmias: any disturbance of the rhythm of the heartbeat.

arteriosclerosis: a pathologic condition of thickening, hardening, or loss of elasticity of the blood vessels, especially arteries, leading to altered function of organs or tissue.

arthritis: inflammation of the joints. *See* Rheumatic disorders.

atony: lack of normal tone, or debility of an organ.

autoimmune: disorder in which the body produces a reaction against itself; allergies and rheumatoid arthritis are examples of autoimmune diseases.

AV block: blockage of the atrioventricular node of the heart causing an abnormal heart rhythm.

bacterial infection: infection due to bacterial causes.
benign prostatic hypertrophy (BPH): swelling of the prostate gland, not caused by cancer. Symptoms usually include increased frequency of urination, increased urination at night, increased difficulty stopping and starting the urinary stream.
biliary: pertaining to the gallbladder.
bowel obstruction: blockage of the intestine.
bradycardia: slow heartbeat.
bronchospasm: tightening of the bronchioles of the lung, causing difficulty breathing.

carcinogen: substance that induces or causes cancer.
celiac disease: a disorder of intestinal malabsorption, which is treated by a diet lacking in gluten, a substance found in wheat and wheat products.
cheilitis: inflammation of the lips or angles of the mouth.
cholecystitis: inflammation of the gallbladder.
cholelithiasis: obstruction of bile flow as a result of a gallstone.
cholestatis: stoppage of bile flow from the gallbladder.
cholinergic: nerve endings which release acetyl-choline, which stimulate the parasympathetic nervous system.
chronic venous insufficiency: inadequate blood flow through the venous system causing swelling and increased risk of clotting, especially to the lower extremities.
CNS: central nervous system, generally pertaining to the brain and spinal column.
colic: spasm, normally of the intestine, causing pain.
colitis: inflammation of the colon.

congestive heart failure: hypertrophy, or swelling of the heart due to lack of blood flow, or as a result of increased work load.

conjunctivitis: inflammation of the conjunctiva, the mucous membranes that line the eyelids.

cor pulmonale: hypertrophy or failure of the right ventricle of the heart from disorders of the lungs or pulmonary vessels.

cystitis: inflammation of the bladder.

dermatitis: inflammation of the skin.

disorder: abnormal condition or disease.

diuretic: substance that causes increased urine flow and decreases edema.

duodenum: the first part of the small intestine connecting with the stomach.

dysmenorrhea: painful menstrual period.

eczema: inflammatory disorder of the skin from numerous causes.

edema: swelling, one of the results of inflammation.

electrolyte: a substance in fluid that conducts electricity; sodium, potassium, chloride, bicarbonate, and calcium are commonly evaluated electrolytes.

emetic: substance that causes vomiting.

enuresis: bedwetting.

envenomation: injection of venom.

erectile dysfunction: inability of the penis to become erect. *See also* Impotence.

esophageal reflux: regurgitation of stomach contents in the esophagus, the muscular tube that extends from the pharynx to the stomach.

essential oil: distillate of a substance.

flatulence: passing gas.

fungal infection: an infection caused by a fungal microorganism.

galactagogue: substance that increases the production of milk.

gastric: pertaining to the stomach.

gastroenteritis: inflammation of the stomach and intestines.

gastrotoxicity: dysfunction of the stomach as a result of a poisonous substance.

gingivitis: inflammation of the gums.

gout: a disorder of excessive uric acid which causes inflammation of the joints.

Graves' disease: swelling of the thyroid gland due to inadequate production of thyroid.

hemorrhoid: mass of swollen veins in the anorectal region.

hemoptysis: coughing up blood.

hepatotoxicity: dysfunction of the liver caused by a poisonous substance.

herpetic: pertaining to herpes virus, such as shingles.

hiatal hernia: a swelling in the opening of the diaphragm where the esophagus passes; often resulting in esophageal reflux.

hypercholesterolemia: elevated levels of cholesterol in the blood. This disorder increases the risk of arteriosclerosis and heart disease.

hypercoagulability: a condition leading to increased clotting of the blood.

hyperemesis gravidarum: excessive vomiting during pregnancy.

hyperhidrosis: excessive sweating.

hyperlipidemia: elevated levels of fat in the blood. This disorder increases the risk of arteriosclerosis and heart disease. Cholesterol and triglycerides are two of the types of lipids found in the blood.

hypertension: elevated blood pressure. This disorder increases the risk of heart disease and/or stroke.

hypertriglyceridemia: elevation of triglyceride, one of the fatty substances in the blood.

hypertrophy: increase in size of an organ or structure not due to a tumor.

hypokalemia: condition of decreased potassium, one of the blood electrolytes.

hypotension: condition of low blood pressure.

immune stimulant: substance that stimulates the immune system.

immunosuppressive: substance that causes, or condition of, decreased immune function.

impotence: inability of the male to copulate.

inflammation: the body's response to stress, including redness, swelling, pain, fever, and decreased function of the tissue or organ. The primary conditions causing inflammation include autoimmune, infectious, traumatic, or cancerous.

insomnia: inability to sleep.

intermittent claudication: condition of decreased blood flow to the lower extremities resulting in extreme pain after walking a specific distance.

intestinal pigmentation: discoloration of the intestine wall, usually caused by certain types of laxatives.

irritable bowel syndrome: common disorder of the colon causing alternating diarrhea and constipation with abdominal pain, or diarrhea alone.

ischemic heart disease: disorder of the heart as a result of decreased blood flow to the heart muscle.

lacrimation: tearing.

lactation: milk production

laxative: substance that causes increased stool.

leukopenia: abnormal decrease in white blood cells.

MAO inhibitors: a class of antidepressant medications.

malaise: discomfort, uneasiness, or indisposition.

mastalgia: pain in the breast.

menorrhagia: excessive bleeding during the menstrual period, either in amount or in number of days.

metrorrhagia: bleeding from the uterus at any time other than during the menstrual period.

mucous membrane: membrane lining passages or cavities which communicate with air; generally refers to the mouth, nose, sinuses, pharynx, rectum, and anus.

multiple sclerosis: Disease of the nervous system that is usually chronic and progressive and characterized by exacerbations and remissions and lesions that are separated in location.

myalgias: pain in the muscles.

myopathy: disorder of the muscles.

NSAIDs: nonsteroidal anti-inflammatory drugs. Medication to decrease inflammation such as Naprosyn or ibuprofen, not of the steroid class of drugs.

nephrotoxicity: dysfunction of the kidney caused by a poisonous substance.

neuralgia: nerve pain.

neurotoxicity: dysfunction of the nervous system caused by a poisonous substance.

obstipation: lack of movement, or stasis, of the gastrointestinal tract.

onychomycosis: fungal infection of the toenails or fingernails.

oral drugs: medication taken by mouth.

palpitations: noticeable abnormal rapid heartbeat.

parasympathetic nervous system: the part of the nervous system that regulates the normal or calm state of the organs.

pharyngitis: inflammation of the pharynx or the back of the throat.

phenothiazine: a type of tranquilizer.

pheochromocytoma: tumor of the adrenal gland causing intermittent adrenaline stimulation.

photosensitivity: inflammatory reaction, usually of skin, to light, especially sunlight.

premenstrual syndrome: bloating, pain, or irritability prior to the menstrual period.

pseudoaldosteronism: abnormal regulatory function of electrolyte balance, not due to the hormone aldosterone. It can occur with chronic licorice overdose.

psoriasis: chronic inflammatory disorder of the skin characterized by silvery-scaled red or pink spots on the skin. Often associated with arthritis.

psychosis: mental disorder of significant severity such that there is a loss of contact with reality.

Raynaud's disease: a disorder of the blood vessel that causes severe spasm to cold or other triggers which decrease the circulation in the peripheral extremities.

renal: pertaining to the kidney.

renal stones: kidney stones.

retinopathy: abnormality of the retina of the eye; frequently associated with chronic diabetes.

rheumatic disorder: abnormal condition of the joints, muscles, and associated structures.

rhinitis: inflammation of the nose.

rhinorrhea: watery discharge from the nose; a runny nose.

seborrhea: disorder of increased production of fatty secretions of the skin.

sedation: process of decreasing nervousness or anxiety; calming, causing sleep.

shingles: inflammation of the skin as a result of herpes virus. Usually on the trunk along a specific nerve pathway.

sinusitis: inflammation of the sinuses.

splenic disorders: conditions or diseases of the spleen.

splenomegaly: enlargement of the spleen.

stasis: lack of movement.

stomatitis: inflammation of the mouth.

stupor: condition of unconsciousness.

sympathetic nervous system: the part of the nervous system that regulates the reaction to stressful stimulus; the "flight or fight" reaction.

tachycardia: rapid heartbeat.

tincture: diluted solution of a substance, usually with alcohol.

tinia pedis: fungal infection of the toes and feet, athlete's foot.

tinnitus: ringing in the ears.

topical: local, usually pertaining to the skin.

trachoma: chronic, contagious conjunctivitis that is viral in origin.

tumor: a swelling or an enlargement; a growth. Can be cancerous or noncancerous.

ulcer: open lesion of the skin or mucous membrane.

upper respiratory infection: infection of the bronchioles of the lung, such as bronchitis or a "cold."

urinary tract infection: infection of the ureters, bladder, or urethra.

urticaria: itching.

utero: in the uterus, pregnancy.

vaginitis: inflammation of the vagina.

varicosities: swelling or twisting of the veins.

vasculitis: inflammation of the blood vessels.

venereal disease: sexually transmitted disease.

vertigo: dizziness.

viral infection: an infection caused by a virus.

xerostomia: decreased salivation, dry mouth.

*I*ndex to Plant Names

Absinth (see ***Artemisia spp.***)   19

Acanthopanax senticosus (see ***Eleutherococcus senticosus***)   56

Achillea millefolium (yarrow, milfoil, nosebleed plant, plumajillo, wound wort)   1

Actaea spp. (white cohosh, baneberry, bugbane, herb Christopher, toad root)   2

Adder's tongue (see ***Stellaria media***)   156

Aesculus hippocastanum (horse chestnut, chestnut, buckeye, Spanish chestnut, common horse chestnut)   3

African coffee tree (see ***Ricinus communis***)   135

African myrrh (see ***Commiphora molmal***)   43

African plum tree (see ***Pygeum africanum***)   128

Agrimonia eupatoria (agrimony, cockleburr, church steeples, common agrimony, sticklewort, stickwort)   4

Agrimony (see ***Agrimonia eupatoria***)   4

Agueweed (see ***Eupatorium perfoliatum***)   60

Ajo (see ***Allium sativum***)   6

Alant (see ***Inula helenium***)   80

Alfalfa (see ***Medicago sativa***)   93

All-heal (see ***Prunella vulgaris*** and ***Valeriana spp.*** and ***Viscum album***)   127, 179, 185

Allium cepa (onion, green onion)   5

Allium sativum (garlic, ajo, poor man's treacle, stinking rose)   6

Allspice (see ***Pimenta spp.***)   114

Aloe spp. (aloe, Barbados aloe, cape aloe)   7

Altamisa (see ***Tanacetem parthenium***)   161

Althea officinalis (marshmallow, mortification root, sweetweed)   8

Amantilla (see ***Valeriana spp.***)   179

Amaranth (see ***Amaranthus spp.***)   9

Amaranthus spp. (amaranth, lady bleeding, love-lies-bleeding, pigweed, pilewort, prince's feather, red cockscomb, velvet flower)   9

Matricaria recutita (chamomile, *Chamomilla recutita*, *Matricaria chamomilla*, German chamomile, Hungarian chamomile, wild chamomile, true chamomile, matricaria)   92

Medicago sativa (alfalfa, buffalo herb, Lucerne, purple medic, purple medick, purple medical)   93

Melaleuca alternifolia (tea tree oil, Australian tea tree oil)   94

Melissa officinalis (lemon balm, balm, sweet balm)   95

Mentha arvensis (mint oil, corn mint oil, field mint oil, Japanese mint oil, marsh mint oil)   96

Mentha piperita (peppermint, brandy mint, lamb mint)   97

Mentha pulegium (pennyroyal, American pennyroyal, European pennyroyal, lurk-in-the-ditch, mosquito plant, pudding plant, squaw balm, squaw mint, tick weed, *Hedeoma pulegioides*)   98

Mentha spicata (spearmint, curled mint, fish mint, garden mint, green mint, lamb mint, mackeral mint, our lady's mint, sage of Bethlehem, yerba buena)   99

Oats (see *Avena sativa*) 22

Ocimum basilicum (basil, common basil, garden basil, holy basil, Saint Joseph's wort, sweet basil) 105

Oenothera spp. (evening primrose, flor-de-Santa Rita, king-cure-all) 106

Oil plant (see *Ricinus communis*) 135

Old woman's broom (see *Turnera diffusa*) 171

Omicha (see *Schisandra chinensis*) 147

One-berry (see *Mitchella spp.*) 100

Oneseed (see *Crataegus monogyra*) 48

Onion (see *Allium cepa*) 5

Orange grape root (see *Berberis spp.*) 24

Orange milkweed (see *Asclepias spp.*) 20

Orange root (see *Hydrastis canadensis*) 76

Oregano (see *Origanum vulgare*) 107

Origano (see *Origanum vulgare*) 107

Origanum vulgare (oregano, European oregano, mountain mint, origano, wild marjoram, winter marjoram, winter sweet) 107

Orris root (see *Iris spp.*) 81

Osier (see *Cornus florida*) 47

Oswego tea (see *Monarda spp.*) 101

Our lady's keys (see *Primula veris*) 126

Our lady's mint (see *Mentha spicata*) 99

Our lady's tea (see *Convallaria majalis*) 45

Ox's tongue (see *Borago officinalis*) 26

Oxlip (see *Primula veris*) 126

Paddock pipes (see *Equisetum arvense*) 58

Paigle (see *Primula veris*) 126

Paigle peggle (see *Primula veris*) 126

Pale gentian (see *Gentiana lutea*) 68

Palma Christi (see *Ricinus communis*) 135

Palsywort (see *Primula veris*) 126

Panang cinnamon (see *Cinnamomum camphora*) 40

Vaccinium macrocarpon (cranberry, *Vaccinium oxycoccos, Vaccinium erythrocarpum, Vaccinium vitis, Vaccinium edule, Vaccinium palustre*)   177

Vaccinium myrtillus (bilberry, *Myrtillus fructus*, bog bilberry, whortle berry, huckleberry, European blue berry)   178

Vaccinium oxycoccos (see ***Vaccinium macrocarpon***)   177

Vaccinium palustre (see ***Vaccinium macrocarpon***)   177

Vaccinium vitis (see ***Vaccinium macrocarpon***)   177

Valerian (see ***Valeriana spp.***)   179

Valeriana edulis (see ***Valeriana spp.***)   179

Valeriana spp. (valerian, *Valeriana edulis*, heliotrope, all-heal, garden valerian, Indian valerian, Mexican valerian, amantilla)   179

Vegetable antimony (see ***Eupatorium perfoliatum***)   60

Velvet flower (see ***Amaranthus spp.***)   9

Veratro verde (see ***Veratrum viride***)   181

Veratrum viride (hellebore, American veratrum, American white hellebore, bugbane, devil's bite, earth gall, false hellebore, green hellebore, green veratrum, Indian poke, itchweed, tickleweed, veratro verde)   181

Verbascum spp. (mullien, blanket lead, bunny ears, candle wick, flannel mullien, large-flowered mullien, Jacob's staff, torch weed, velvet plant)   182

Verbena spp. (vervain, blue vervain, common verbena, common vervain, enchanter's plant, European vervain, herb of grace, herb of the cross, holywort, Juon's tears, pigeon's grass, pigeonweed, simpler's joy, turkey grass)   183

Vervain (see ***Verbena spp.***)   183

Viburnum (see ***Viburnum prunifolium***)   184

Viburnum prunifolium (black haw, American sloe, European cranberry, crampbark, dog rowan tree, guelder rose, king's crown, high cranberry, may rose, nanny berry, red elder, rose elder, wheep berry, shonny, silver bells, sloe, snowball tree, southern black haw, stag bush, viburnum, water elder, whitsun bosses)   184

*I*ndex to Indications

INDEX TO INDICATIONS

INDEX TO INDICATIONS

► INDEX TO INDICATIONS

*I*ndex to Contraindications

Note: Avoidance of use of herbal remedies in children, during lactation, or pregnancy is listed when that specific contraindication is substantiated in reference texts. Use of herbal remedies in any of these situations must be carefully weighed against the risk.

Antithrombotic agents (anticoagulants, antiplatelets, aspirin)

*I*ndex to Potential
Medication Interactions